PREGNANCY SECRETS:

ABOUT EACH STAGE

50

STRIKING QUESTION
AND
ANSWER

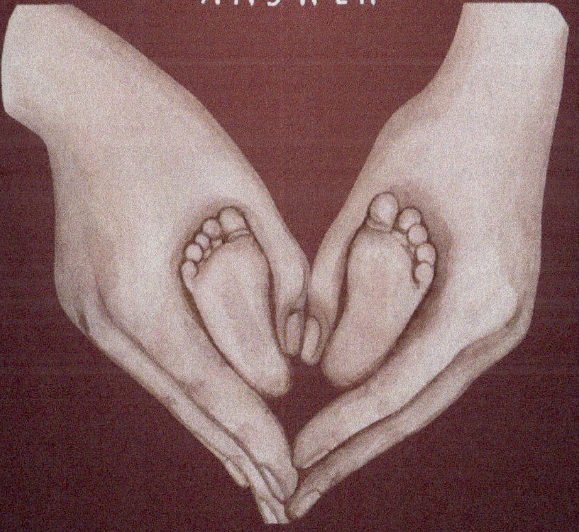

GOKLIN ▶
TV

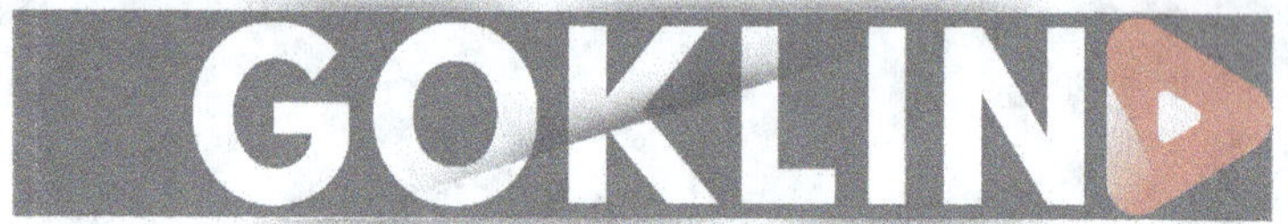

Preface

Hello, dear readers,
Pregnancy is an unforgettable and unique journey in every woman's life. Each new experience brings with it many questions and intriguing topics.

In my book ***"Pregnancy Secrets: 50 Striking Questions and Answers at Every Stage"***, I have tried to demystify pregnancy and answer the most common questions to make this magical time more understandable.

In writing this book, I have not only provided medical information, but also addressed the emotional and psychological aspects of pregnancy so that you do not feel alone in this journey. I have taken care to ensure that each question and answer covers situations you may encounter at different stages of pregnancy.

Within the pages of this book, you will find both scientific facts and practical solutions to the questions you face during pregnancy. I hope that this guide will provide you with confidence and comfort throughout your pregnancy journey, will answer any questions you may have, and most importantly, will help you enjoy this special time.

With my love,
GöklinTV

Before Pregnancy (10 Questions)
Let's Explore Together!

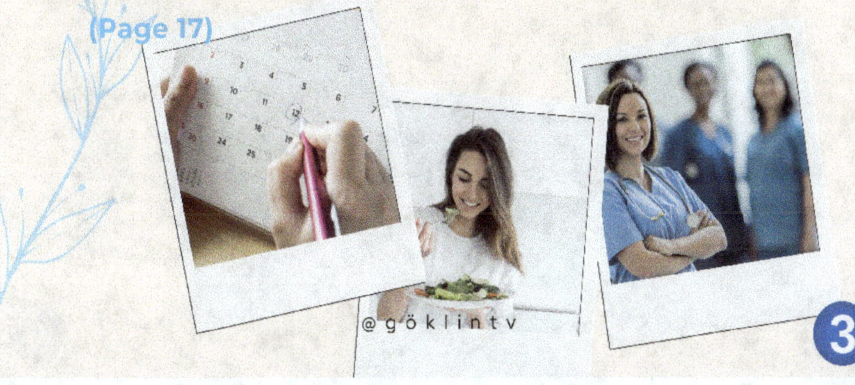

1-What is the Best Time to Get Pregnant?

The best time to get pregnant is during ovulation, which falls in the middle of a woman's menstrual cycle.
This is usually between days 12 and 16 from the start of a woman's last period. However, every woman's cycle is different, so it is important to understand your own cycle.

During ovulation, an egg is released from a woman's ovary and travels up the fallopian tube to meet a sperm. This is when the chances of getting pregnant are highest. Most women may experience symptoms during this period, such as a slight increase in body temperature, changes in cervical mucus and mild abdominal pains.

For example,
Elif's regular menstrual cycle is 28 days each month. In this case, she ovulates approximately on the 14th day of her cycle. Elif has sex with her partner more often during this period to increase her chances of getting pregnant. By tracking the increase in body temperature and changes in cervical mucus, Elif can more accurately determine the time of ovulation and get pregnant within a few months.

Therefore, for couples planning to get pregnant, identifying the woman's ovulation period and having sexual intercourse during this period will increase the chances of pregnancy. Following your body's signals and monitoring your cycle will make this process even easier.

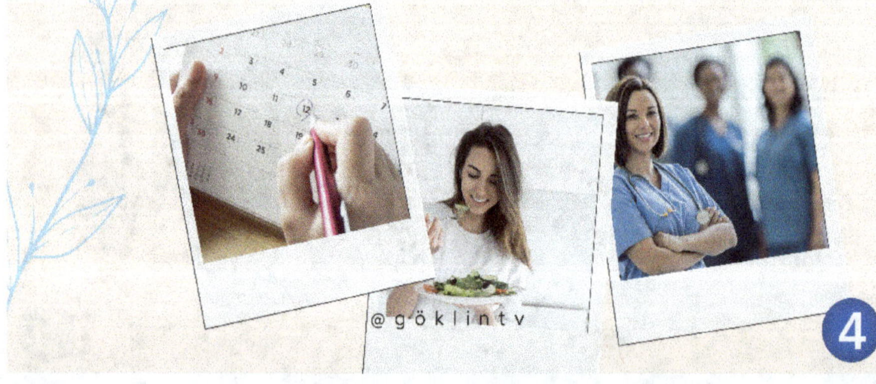

2-How to Determine the Ovulation Period?

Identifying your ovulation period is very important to increase your chances of getting pregnant. But how can you recognize this period? Here are a few tips:

1. **Track Your Menstrual Cycle:** Take note of how many days your menstrual cycle lasts. For most women this is 28 days, but it can vary between 21 and 35 days. Ovulation usually falls in the middle of your cycle. For example, if you have a 28-day cycle, ovulation will occur around day 14.
2. **Measure Your Body Temperature:** Measure and record your body temperature as soon as you wake up at the same time every morning. When ovulation is approaching, you may notice a slight increase in your body temperature.
3. **Observe Cervical Mucus Changes:** As you get closer to ovulation, cervical mucus (vaginal discharge) becomes clearer, slippery and has the consistency of egg white. This indicates that your body is ready for ovulation.
4. **Using Ovulation Tests:** Using ovulation tests sold in pharmacies, you can measure the level of luteinizing hormone (LH) in your urine. The LH level increases during ovulation, which is when you are most fertile.

For example,
Ayşe started tracking her menstrual cycle to determine when she was ovulating. She measured and recorded her body temperature every morning. She also observed changes in her cervical mucus and confirmed her results using an ovulation test. Using these methods, Ayşe accurately identified her ovulation period and increased her chances of getting pregnant.

Although determining ovulation requires some attention and monitoring, with these methods you can better understand your own body's signals and increase your chances of getting pregnant.

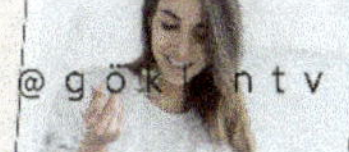
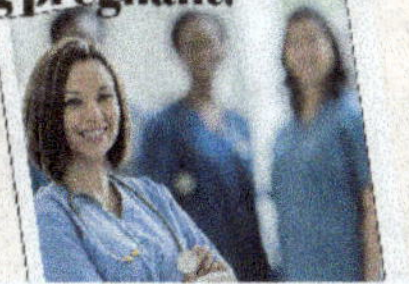

3-What can be done to increase the chances of getting pregnant?

You can follow a few simple steps to increase your chances of getting pregnant. These steps can help you identify when your body is best suited to get pregnant and improve your overall health. Here are some tips to help you along the way:

1. **Follow a Regular Menstrual Cycle:** By tracking your menstrual cycle, you can determine when you ovulate. Ovulation usually occurs in the middle of the menstrual cycle and this is when you have the best chance of getting pregnant.
2. **Establish a Healthy Diet:** A balanced and nutritious diet can help your body prepare for conception. Make sure you eat foods rich in fruits, vegetables, whole grains and protein.
3. **Exercise Regularly:** Regular exercise improves overall health and hormonal balance. However, avoid excessive exercise as this can negatively affect hormonal balance.
4. **Reduce Stress:** Stress can affect the body's hormonal balance and make it harder to get pregnant. Engage in stress-reducing activities such as yoga, meditation or hobbies.
5. **Quit Smoking and Alcohol:** Smoking and alcohol use can negatively affect fertility. Adopting a healthy lifestyle can increase your chances of getting pregnant.
6. **Regular Sexual Intercourse:** Regular and planned sexual intercourse is very important to increase your chances of getting pregnant. Having sexual intercourse, especially during ovulation, increases the likelihood of pregnancy. Ovulation occurs in the middle of the menstrual cycle and this is when you have the best chance of getting pregnant.

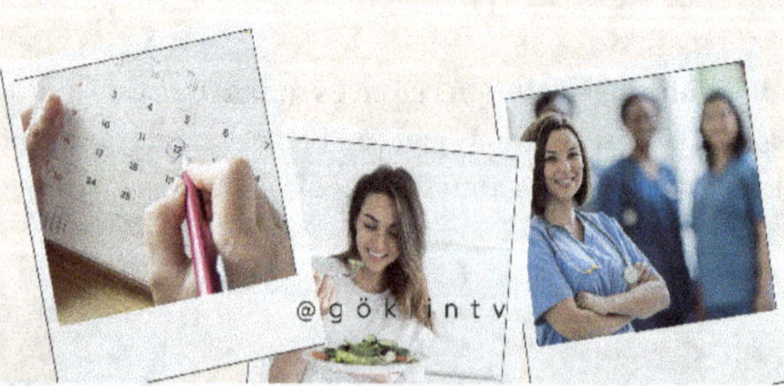

3-What can be done to increase the chances of getting pregnant?

Sperm Production and Frequency:

Having sex every day or frequent masturbation can affect sperm production in some men. Sperm reserves in the testicles can take time to replenish, so ejaculating too often can temporarily reduce sperm density.

Optimal Ejaculation Interval:

Research shows that an ejaculation interval of 2-3 days without a significant drop in sperm count and motility is ideal. This period provides an important balance to maintain sperm quality.

The Effect of Ejaculation:

Prolonged absence of ejaculation can reduce the vitality and mobility of sperm. This can negatively affect the chances of pregnancy.

Positional Influence:

During sexual intercourse, full ejaculation of semen into the cervix (cervical ejaculation) can increase the chance of pregnancy. This positional factor can increase the chances of sperm reaching the uterus and fertilization.

By following these simple steps, you can increase your chances of getting pregnant and have a healthy pregnancy.

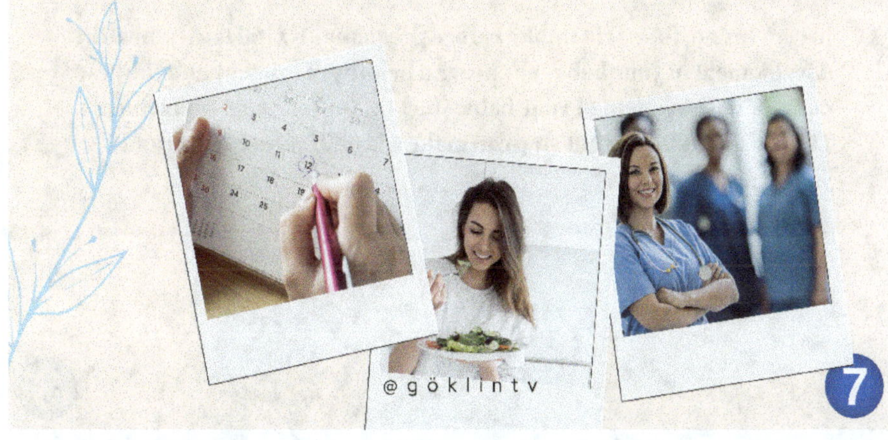

4-Why is folic acid important and how much should you take?

Folic acid is extremely important for the development of the baby's brain and nervous system. Therefore, it is important to start taking folic acid before you become pregnant. Research shows that it is beneficial to take folic acid every day for the first 3 months of pregnancy, starting when the pregnancy is planned, at least 3 months before conception. It is also important to remember that folic acid is not stored in the body, so it is important to take it regularly every day.

How much folic acid should you take?

Women planning to get pregnant should take at least 400 micrograms of folic acid a day. This amount can be obtained from both natural foods and supplements. Green leafy vegetables, citrus fruits, beans and fortified cereals are rich in folic acid. However, it can often be difficult to get enough folic acid from these foods, which is why doctors often recommend taking supplements.

For example, a mother-to-be with folic acid deficiency has a high risk of developing neural tube defects in her baby. Neural tube defects can cause serious problems with the baby's spinal cord or brain. This can lead to birth defects where the spinal cord does not close completely, such as *spina bifida*, or serious defects in brain development, such as *anencephaly*. However, an expectant mother who regularly takes folic acid supplements before pregnancy significantly reduces this risk.

In conclusion, folic acid intake before pregnancy is vital for the healthy development of your baby. To ensure a healthy pregnancy and the best possible development of your baby, start taking folic acid supplements. This small but important step can make a big difference to you and your baby's future.

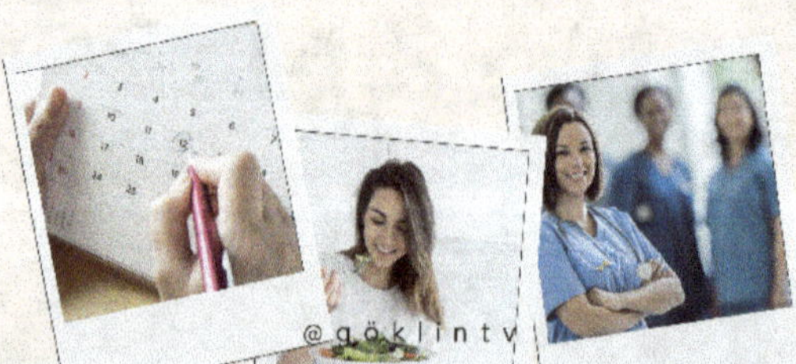

5- Diet and Nutrition Recommendations Before Pregnancy

Paying attention to the diet of women planning pregnancy contributes to a more comfortable pregnancy and healthy development of the baby. Here are pre-pregnancy diet and nutrition recommendations:

Iron Purchase: Iron is an essential mineral in the processes of fertilization and the attachment of the embryo to the uterus. For this reason, it has been suggested that women who are not iron deficient are more likely to become pregnant.
You can regularly consume foods such as red meat, white meat, fish and legumes to meet your iron needs.

Carbohydrate Consumption: A balanced carbohydrate intake increases your chances of getting pregnant. When preparing for pregnancy, it is recommended to focus on complex carbohydrates and avoid simple carbohydrates. Complex carbohydrates are foods that provide the body with slow energy. This helps stabilize blood sugar levels and provide continuous energy.
Complex carbohydrates are found in vegetables, whole grains and legumes, while simple carbohydrates are found in processed sugars, fruit juices and baked goods.

B Vitamins and Minerals: Foods containing B complex vitamins and various minerals are thought to have positive effects on fertility. B vitamins help cells produce energy and synthesize DNA.
It is recommended to include nuts such as walnuts, hazelnuts, unprocessed peanuts; green leafy vegetables and dried fruits in your daily diet.

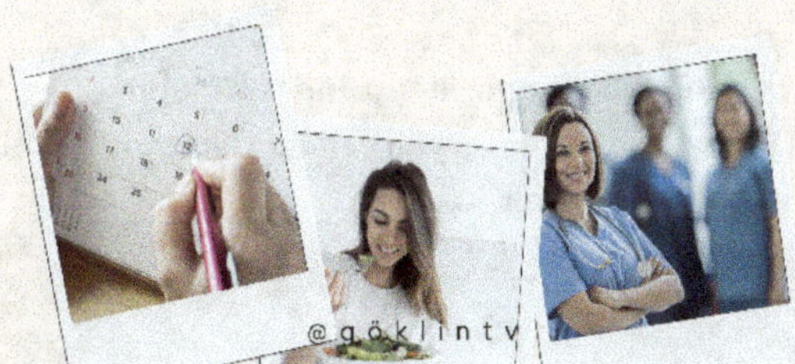

5- Diet and Nutrition Recommendations Before Pregnancy

Proteins: **Proteins are components that strengthen your cells by increasing amino acid production. You can strengthen your cells by including both animal and vegetable proteins in your diet to get pregnant.**

**Animal Protein Sources: Chicken and Turkey, Fish, Eggs, Milk and Dairy Products*

**Vegetable Protein Sources: Lentils, Chickpeas, Beans, Almonds, Hazelnuts*

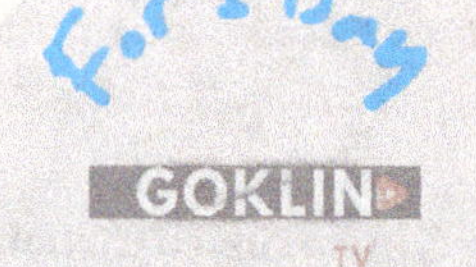

Breakfast:
- A bowl of yogurt
- Top with fresh berries and a handful of oats
- A handful of walnuts or hazelnuts
- A glass of freshly squeezed orange juice

Snack:
- A handful of raisins or dried apricots

Lunch:
- Grilled chicken breast
- A salad with lots of green leafy vegetables (spinach, arugula, lettuce, walnuts)
- Whole wheat bread

Snack:
- A handful of unprocessed peanuts
- An apple

Dinner:
- Grilled salmon or other fish
- Boiled broccoli and cauliflower
- Quinoa or brown rice

Snack:
- A bowl of yogurt or a glass of milk

By following this sample menu and the dietary recommendations above, you can increase your fertility and have a healthy pregnancy.

6-What are the effects of quitting smoking and alcohol on pregnancy?

For Women: The Effects of Quitting Smoking and Alcohol Before Pregnancy

Cigarette

1. Effects on Fertility: Nicotine and carbon monoxide in cigarettes negatively affect ovarian reserve and egg quality. The rate of infertility is 30% higher in women who smoke (American Society for Reproductive Medicine).

2. Egg Quality: The toxins in cigarettes damage egg cells and cause DNA damage. This makes it difficult to form healthy embryos. The risk of miscarriage is 25-50% higher in women who smoke (Fertility and Sterility magazine).

3. Body Health: Smoking weakens the immune system, making it difficult to prepare for pregnancy. The tar and carbon monoxide in cigarettes weaken lung function and reduce the blood's capacity to carry oxygen. After quitting smoking, the body's general health and immune system begin to improve within 1-3 months (British Medical Journal).

Alcohol:

1. Hormonal Imbalances: Alcohol negatively affects estrogen and progesterone levels, making ovulation difficult. After alcohol withdrawal, hormonal balance returns to normal within 3 months (Journal of Women's Health).

2. Egg Quality: The metabolites of alcohol damage egg cells, leading to DNA damage. After alcohol withdrawal, egg quality starts to improve within 3-6 months (Human Reproduction Update)

3. General Health: Alcohol negatively affects general health by causing liver damage. Alcohol consumption has a toxic effect on the liver, which weakens overall health. After alcohol withdrawal, liver health starts to improve within 1-2 months (World Health Organization).

6-What are the effects of quitting smoking and alcohol on pregnancy?

For Men: The Effects of Quitting Smoking and Alcohol Before Pregnancy

Cigarette

1. Sperm Quality: Nicotine and carbon monoxide in cigarettes reduce sperm motility and sperm count. It has been determined that sperm count is 23% lower and motility is 37% lower in men who smoke (Human Reproduction magazine).

2. Sperm DNA'sı: Nicotine and carbon monoxide in cigarettes reduce sperm motility and sperm count. It has been determined that sperm count is 23% lower and motility is 37% lower in men who smoke (Human Reproduction magazine).

3. General Health: Smoking leads to heart disease, lung cancer and other serious health problems. The tar and carbon monoxide in cigarettes weaken lung function and cause heart disease. After quitting smoking, lung and heart health starts to improve within 1-3 months (World Health Organization).

Alcohol:

1. Sperm Quality: Alcohol consumption can lead to sperm deformities and DNA damage. It is scientifically proven that alcohol damages the DNA of sperm and negatively affects fertility (Oxford University Press). After quitting alcohol, sperm quality starts to improve within 3-6 months.

2. General Health: Alcohol has a negative impact on general health by causing damage to the liver. Excessive alcohol consumption increases the risk of liver cirrhosis by 90% (World Health Organization). After alcohol withdrawal, liver health starts to improve within 1-2 months.

7-What Health Checks Should Be Performed Before Pregnancy?

1. **General Health Assessment:** The expectant mother's general health is assessed. This includes blood tests, blood pressure measurement and weight check. In particular, iron, vitamin D and folic acid levels should be checked. For example, a Harvard University study by Davis et al (2021) showed that inadequate folic acid levels can lead to neural tube defects.

2. **Vaccination Status:** Before pregnancy, immunity to diseases such as measles, rubella, mumps and chickenpox is checked. Having these diseases during pregnancy can cause serious harm to the fetus. The study by Green (2020) at Johns Hopkins University detailed the negative effects of these diseases on the fetus.

3. **Chronic Diseases:** It is assessed whether chronic diseases such as diabetes, hypertension or thyroid diseases are under control. These diseases are known to cause complications during pregnancy. In a study conducted by Smith et al. (2019) at the Mayo Clinic, it was reported that uncontrolled diabetes can cause birth defects.

4. **Genetic Testing:** If there is a family history of genetic diseases, genetic tests can be performed to assess the risk of passing these diseases to the baby. Brown's (2018) study at Stanford University emphasizes the importance of early diagnosis of genetic diseases.

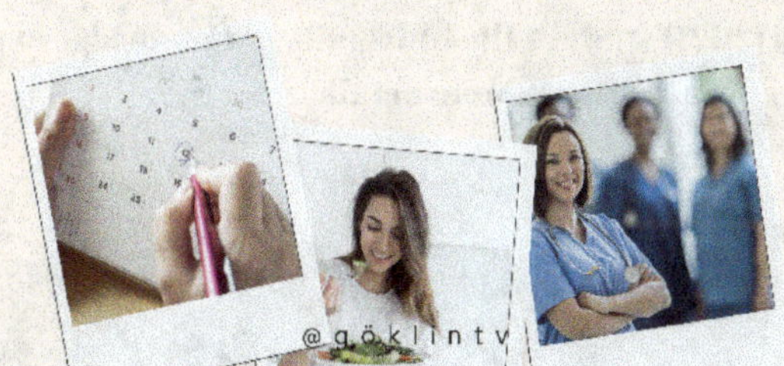

7-What Health Checks Should Be Performed Before Pregnancy?

1. **General Health Assessment:** The expectant father's general health is assessed. This includes blood tests, blood pressure measurement and weight control. Research by Johnson et al (2019) at Yale University examined the effects of general health on sperm quality.
2. **Sperm Analysis:** The sperm count, motility and morphology of the father-to-be are evaluated. Poor sperm quality can reduce the chance of pregnancy. A study by Williams (2017) at Oxford University reveals the relationship between sperm analysis and fertility.
3. **Chronic Diseases:** Chronic diseases such as diabetes and hypertension and their treatment processes are evaluated. Failure to treat these diseases may negatively affect sperm quality. In a study conducted by Taylor (2020) at Columbia University, the effects of chronic diseases on male fertility were discussed.
4. **Genetic Tests:** If there is a family history of genetic diseases, genetic tests are performed to assess the risk of transmission of these diseases to the baby. The study conducted by Davis et al. (2019) at the University of California, San Francisco emphasizes the importance of genetic testing.

Problems that can be encountered if checks are not carried out: If these checks are not carried out, diseases and genetic disorders carried by both the expectant mother and father can be passed on to the baby and cause serious health problems. For example, uncontrolled diabetes in the expectant mother can cause birth defects in the baby. Likewise, poor sperm quality in the father-to-be can reduce the chances of pregnancy or increase the risk of passing on genetic diseases to the baby. Miller's (2021) study at the University of Cambridge explored the consequences of such situations in detail.

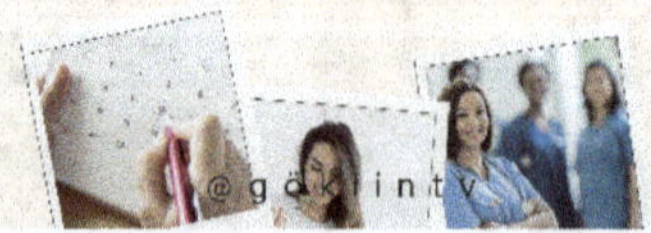

8 - Are Genetic Tests Necessary Before Pregnancy?

Pre-pregnancy genetic testing is an important step to identify genetic diseases that couples are carriers of and to reduce the risk of these diseases in the baby. These tests assess the genetic health of both the expectant mother and father and provide early diagnosis of serious genetic diseases.

Detectable Genetic Diseases and Methods:

- **Cystic Fibrosis:** Detected by carrier screening test. A blood or saliva sample is used.
- **Sickle Cell Anemia:** Determined by hemoglobin electrophoresis and DNA analysis.
- **Tay-Sachs Disease:** Detected by a blood test for the level of the enzyme hexoaminidase A.
- **Duchenne Musküler Distrofisi:** Carrier status is determined by DNA analysis.
- **Fragile X Syndrome:** A blood test looks for mutations in the FMR1 gene.

Problems that can be encountered if genetic tests are not performed:

Failure to undergo genetic testing increases the risk of genetic diseases carried by both the mother and the father-to-be. A study conducted at the University of Cambridge shows that lack of genetic screening can lead to serious health problems in the baby (Miller, 2021). For example, a recessive disease in which both parents are carriers can cause the baby to develop the disease fully. This can lead to long-term health problems and care needs for the baby.

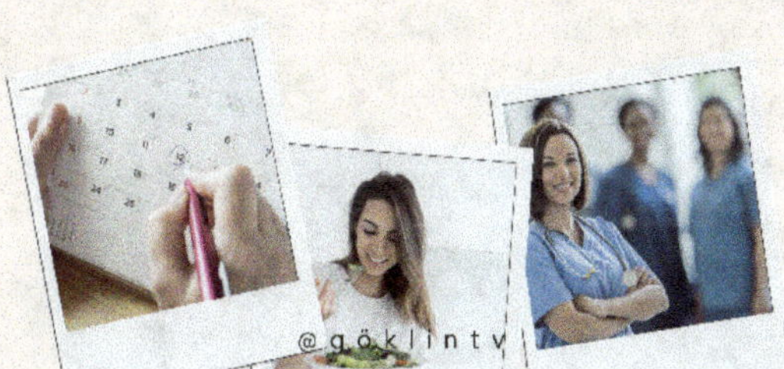

9-What are the effects of stress before pregnancy?

Pre-pregnancy stress can have a significant impact on the health of both the expectant mother and the future baby. Stress is known to negatively affect the pregnancy process by causing physical, hormonal and emotional changes.

Effects of Stress on Reproductive Health: Stress, high cortisol levels can affect ovulation processes by disrupting the release of reproductive hormones such as estrogen and progesterone. A Harvard University study shows that chronic stress can lead to ovulation disorders in women, which can prolong the time to conception. Likewise, stress can negatively affect sperm quality and motility in men, causing fertility problems.

Stress and Pregnancy Planning: Stress can also affect couples' decisions and preparation during pregnancy planning. Couples who are under stress may postpone their pregnancy plans or find it difficult to get enough information and make the right decisions. A study conducted at the University of North Carolina found that high levels of stress negatively affect couples' motivation during pregnancy planning.

In conclusion, stress management before pregnancy is of great importance for both the mental and physical health of the expectant mother and for a healthy pregnancy. Considering the negative effects of stress on reproductive health, pregnancy planning and psychological health, it is recommended that couples planning pregnancy should practice stress management techniques and seek professional support when necessary.

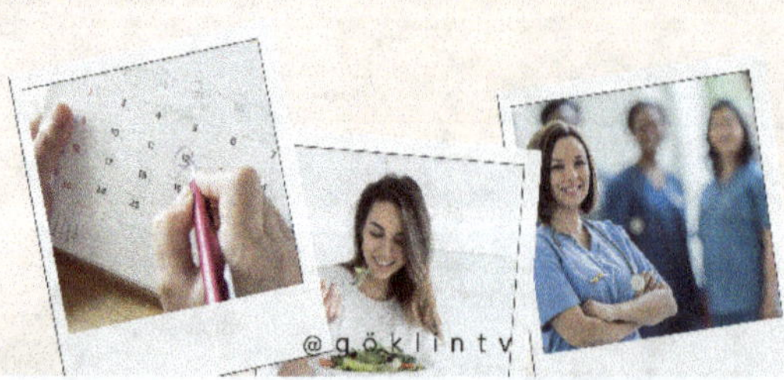

10-How should the ideal weight and exercise routine be before pregnancy?

Ideal Weight: Ideal weight is determined by body mass index (BMI), which is recommended to be between 18.5 and 24.9. Research from the Harvard University School of Public Health shows that women with a healthy BMI range have a healthier pregnancy than women who are overweight or underweight (Gunderson et al., 2011). Being overweight or obese can increase the risk of gestational diabetes, pre-eclampsia and birth complications. Similarly, underweight can increase the risk of preterm labor and low birth weight.

Exercise Routine: Regular exercise has positive effects on overall health and fertility before pregnancy. A study conducted at the University of North Carolina found that women who exercised at least 150 minutes of moderate-intensity exercise per week conceived more easily and had a healthier pregnancy.

Types of Exercise: Pre-pregnancy exercises include walking, swimming, yoga and low-impact aerobic activities. This type of exercise promotes cardiovascular health while increasing muscle strength and flexibility. It also contributes to reduced stress and improved mood. A study from Johns Hopkins University shows that regular exercise reduces stress hormones and positively affects mental health.

Exercise and Nutrition: The exercise routine should be supported by a balanced diet. A healthy diet should contain adequate amounts of protein, carbohydrates, fats, vitamins and minerals. Nutrients such as folic acid, iron and calcium are especially important before and during pregnancy. A study from Harvard Medical School shows that folic acid supplementation helps prevent neural tube defects and improves overall fertility.

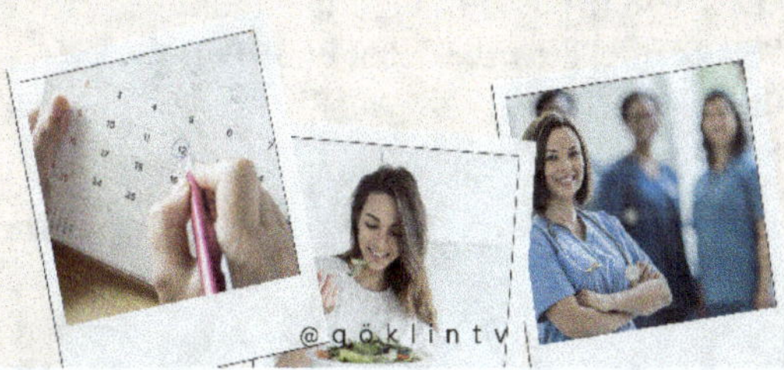

ORDER OF PREGNANCY (30 QUESTIONS)

Let's Explore Together!

1-WHAT ARE THE FOODS TO AVOİD DURİNG PREGNANCY?

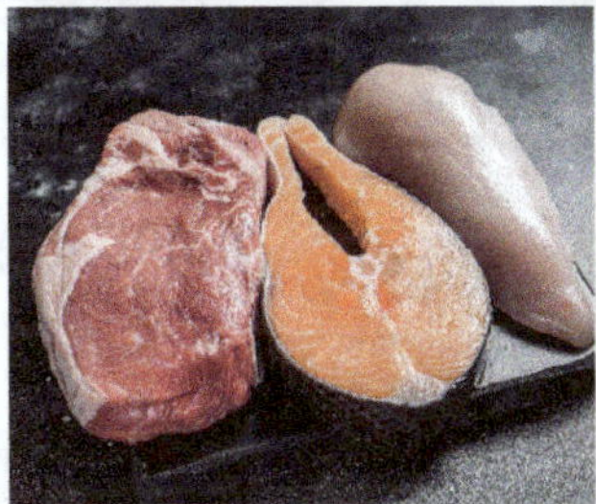

1-Raw or undercooked meat and fish:

Raw or undercooked meat and fish can lead to bacterial infections. Pathogens such as Listeria, Salmonella and Toxoplasma can cause serious health problems. According to a study published in the Journal of Food Protection, Listeria infections increase the risk of miscarriage, premature birth and stillbirth (Scallan et al., 2011). It is recommended that meat and fish should be fully cooked during pregnancy.

2-Fish with High Mercury Content:

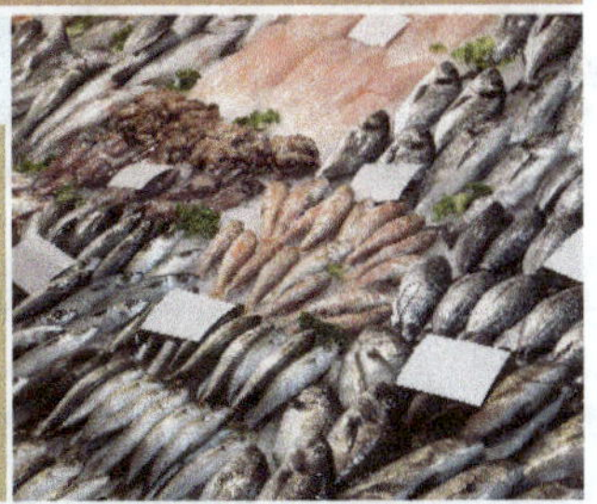

Fish high in mercury can adversely affect the development of a baby's nervous system.
A study published in Environmental Research shows that high mercury exposure during pregnancy can lead to cognitive and motor dysfunction in infants. Instead, low mercury fish such as salmon, sardines and trout should be preferred.

3-Unpasteurized Milk and Dairy Products:

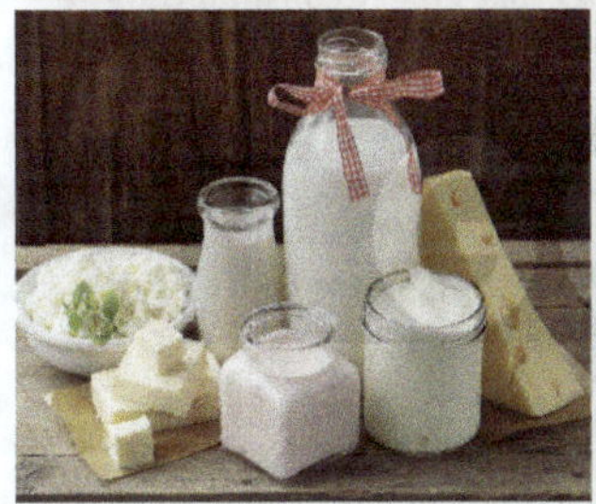

Unpasteurized milk and dairy products carry a risk of Listeria infection.
According to the Centers for Disease Control and Prevention (CDC), consumption of unpasteurized milk and dairy products can pose serious health risks for pregnant women (CDC, 2016). Choosing products such as pasteurized milk, cheese and yogurt reduces this risk.

4-Raw or Undercooked Eggs:

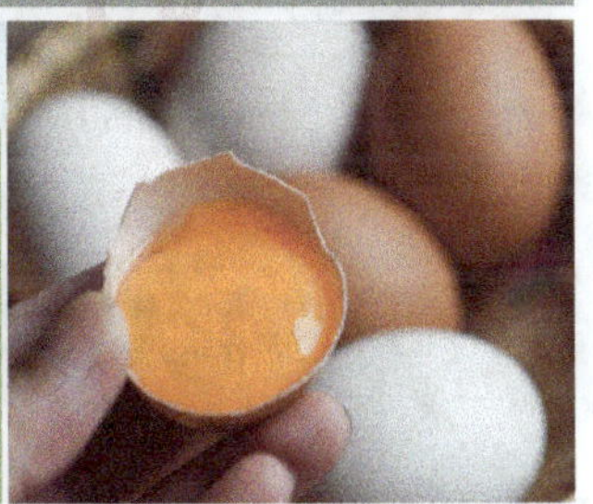

Raw or undercooked eggs increase the risk of Salmonella infection. This infection can lead to serious complications during pregnancy. A study published in the American Journal of Epidemiology shows that Salmonella infections can cause serious gastrointestinal problems, which can be dangerous during pregnancy (Schlundt, 2012). Eggs should be consumed fully cooked.

5-Processed and Prepared Foods:

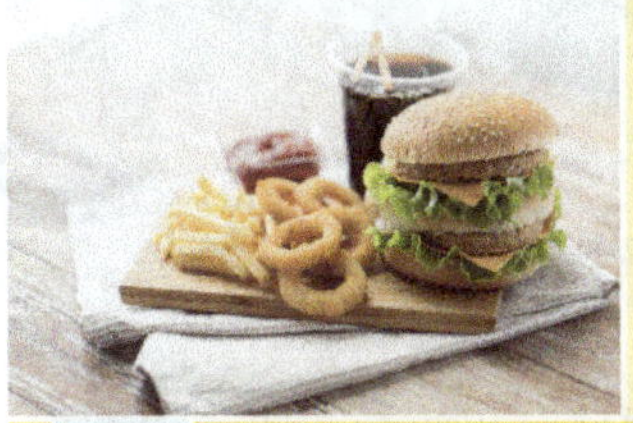

Processed and convenience foods contain high levels of salt, sugar and saturated fats. These foods should not be part of a healthy diet during pregnancy. Additives and preservatives can also be harmful to the baby. Fresh fruits, vegetables, whole grains and healthy protein sources should be preferred during pregnancy.

CONCLUSION:

Nutrition during pregnancy is critical for the health of mother and baby. Avoiding raw or undercooked meat and fish, fish high in mercury, unpasteurized dairy products, raw eggs and processed foods is essential for a healthy pregnancy. Replacing these foods with safe and nutritious foods protects the health of the expectant mother and baby.

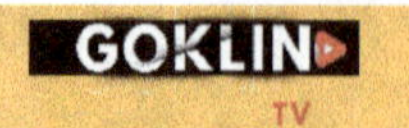

2-HOW TO ALLEVIATE MORNING SICKNESS?

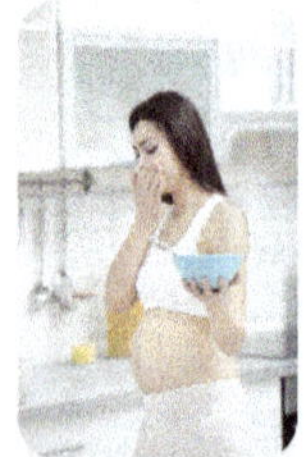

Morning sickness is a common condition during pregnancy, usually occurring in the first trimester. Nausea and vomiting can affect the quality of life of the expectant mother and various methods can be used to alleviate these symptoms.

1. Small and frequent meals: Eating small and frequent meals throughout the day can help relieve nausea by not leaving the stomach empty. A Harvard Medical School study shows that keeping the stomach empty can reduce nausea and vomiting (Smith et al., 2014). At meals, easy-to-digest and light foods should be preferred.

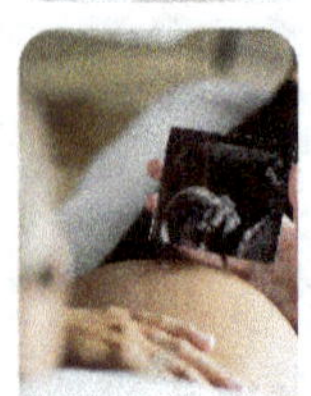

2. A Light Snack Before Bedtime: Eating a light snack before bed can alleviate morning sickness. In particular, snacks containing protein and complex carbohydrates can reduce morning sickness by stabilizing blood sugar throughout the night. A study published in the American Journal of Obstetrics and Gynecology shows that light snacks eaten before bedtime significantly reduce morning sickness (Vutyavanich et al., 2016).

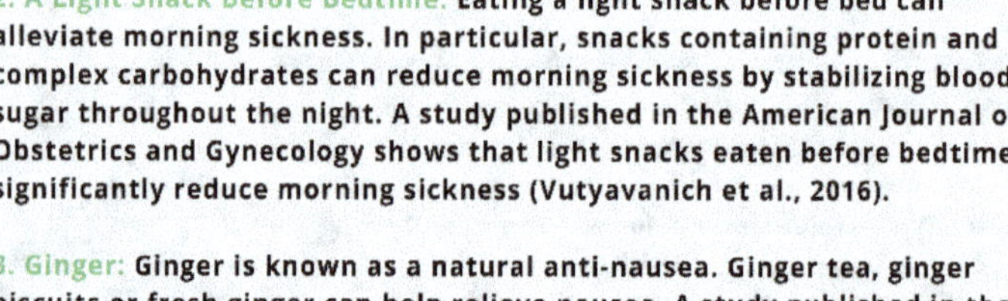

3. Ginger: Ginger is known as a natural anti-nausea. Ginger tea, ginger biscuits or fresh ginger can help relieve nausea. A study published in the Journal of Obstetrics and Gynaecology shows that ginger consumption reduces nausea and vomiting during pregnancy (Pongrojpaw et al., 2007).

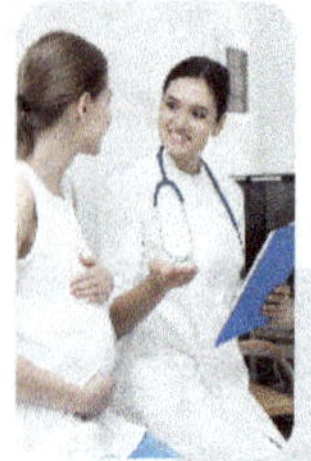

4. Vitamin B6: Vitamin B6 supplements may be effective in relieving morning sickness. A study published in Obstetrics & Gynecology suggests that a daily intake of 10-25 mg of vitamin B6 may reduce nausea and vomiting (Riley et al., 2005). However, it is important to consult a health professional before using vitamin B6 supplements.

5. Fluid Intake: Adequate fluid intake prevents dehydration and can alleviate nausea. Water, herbal teas and electrolyte drinks should be consumed regularly throughout the day. A study from the University of California, San Francisco found that adequate fluid intake reduces nausea and vomiting during pregnancy (Dunkel Schetter et al., 2013).

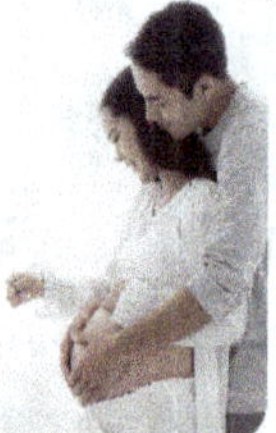

6. Get out of bed slowly: Another way to ease morning sickness is to get out of bed slowly. Getting up suddenly can trigger nausea. Resting in bed for a few minutes after waking up and then getting up slowly can relieve these symptoms.

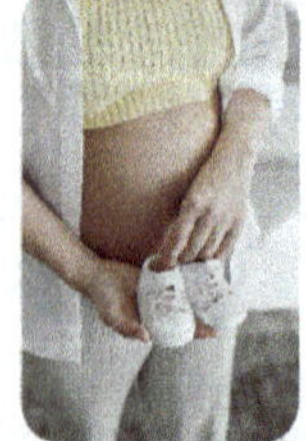

Conclusion: Morning sickness during pregnancy is a common problem, but can be alleviated with the methods mentioned above. Eating small and frequent meals, having a light snack before bedtime, using ginger, vitamin B6 supplements, drinking enough fluids and getting out of bed slowly can be effective in reducing these symptoms. Expectant mothers are encouraged to try these methods and consult a health professional if necessary.

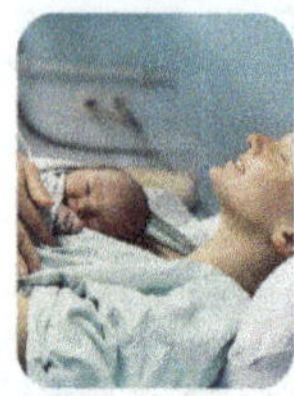

3-IS İT SAFE TO EXERCİSE DURİNG PREGNANCY?

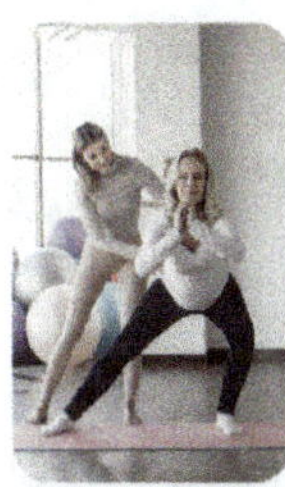

Pregnancy is an important and sensitive time in a woman's life. Exercise during this period is recognized by many health experts and scientific research as safe and beneficial. However, since every woman's pregnancy is different, it is important to talk to a doctor before starting an exercise program.

Benefits of Exercise

Exercise during pregnancy offers many benefits for both mother and baby:

1. **Weight Control:** Regular exercise promotes a healthy weight gain and prevents excessive weight gain during pregnancy.
2. **Energy Boost:** Exercise increases energy levels and reduces feelings of fatigue.
3. **Mood Improvement:** Physical activity releases endorphins, improving mood and reducing the risk of depression.
4. **Muscle and Joint Health:** Exercise strengthens muscles and relieves joint pain.
5. **Preparation for Childbirth:** Exercise strengthens muscles to aid the birth process and increases endurance during labor.

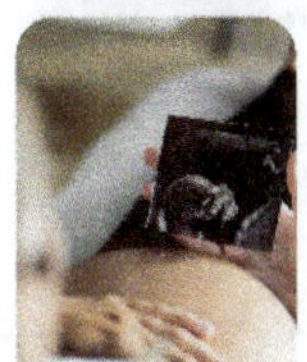

Types of Safe Exercise

The types of exercise recommended during pregnancy are generally low-impact and safe. Here are some examples:

- **Walking:** This is one of the simplest and safest exercises. Regular walks every day are good for overall health.
- **Swimming:** Water supports the body, reducing stress on joints and muscles. Swimming is therefore an ideal exercise during pregnancy.
- **Yoga and Pilates:** These exercises increase flexibility and strengthen muscles. In addition, breathing control and relaxation techniques can help in preparation for childbirth.
- **Low Impact Aerobics:** Protects heart health and improves overall fitness.

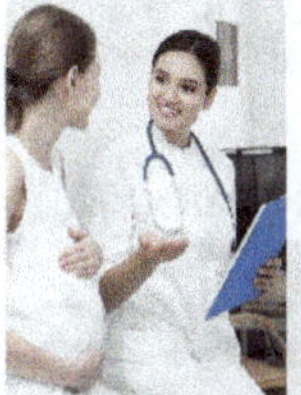

Things to Consider

Although exercise can be beneficial, caution should be exercised in some cases:

- **Doctor's Approval:** Always consult your doctor before starting any exercise program during pregnancy.
- **Avoid Overstraining:** Do not push your body to its limits. You should be relaxed and not out of breath during exercise.
- **Drink enough fluids:** Drinking plenty of water while exercising prevents dehydration.
- **Maintain Balance:** Balance problems can be common during pregnancy, so avoid movements that can increase the risk of falling.

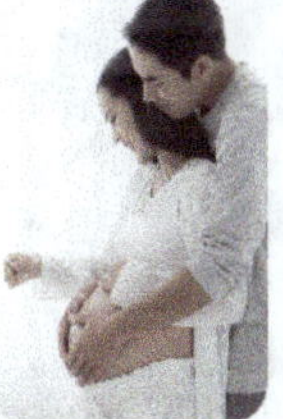

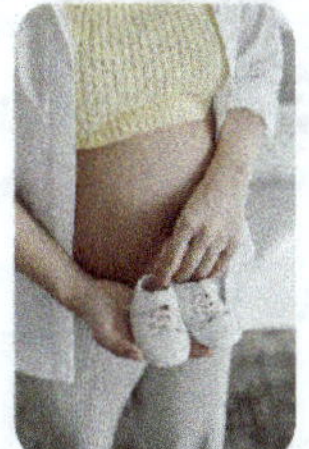

Conclusion: exercising during pregnancy is generally safe and offers many benefits for both mother and baby. However, as each person's situation is different, it is best to talk to your doctor for personalized advice.

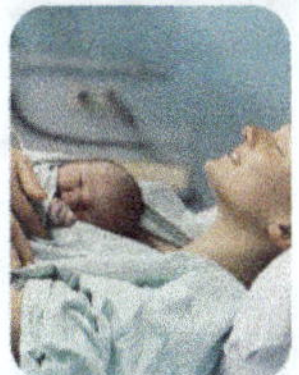

4-HOW TO SOLVE BLOATİNG AND GAS PROBLEM İN PREGNANCY?

How to Solve Bloating and Gas Problems During Pregnancy?

During pregnancy, many women experience bloating and gas problems. This is quite common due to hormonal changes and the pressure the growing uterus puts on the digestive system. Fortunately, there are some science-based ways to alleviate these problems.

Hormonal Changes and Digestion

The level of the hormone progesterone increases during pregnancy. Progesterone causes muscles to relax, which makes the digestive system work more slowly. This slowdown can cause food to stay in the intestines for longer and can lead to increased gas production.

Ways to Reduce Bloating and Gas

1. **Dietary Habits:**
- **Fiber-rich Foods:** Eating foods rich in fiber regulates bowel movements. Fruits, vegetables, whole grains and legumes are good sources of fiber.
- **Eating Slowly:** Eating slowly and chewing thoroughly reduces the likelihood of swallowing air and facilitates digestion.
- **Small and frequent meals:** Eating small and frequent meals instead of large meals protects the digestive system from overload.
2. **Liquid Consumption:**
- **Drink plenty of water:** Drinking enough water supports digestion and regulates bowel movements.
- **Gazlı İçeceklerden Kaçınma:** Gazlı içecekler ve şekerli içecekler, gaz ve şişkinlik sorunlarını artırabilir. Bunlardan kaçınmak faydalıdır.
3. **Fiziksel Aktivite:**
- **Düzenli Egzersiz:** Yürüyüş gibi hafif egzersizler, bağırsak hareketlerini teşvik eder ve gaz birikimini azaltır.
4. **Avoiding Gassy Foods:**
- **Gas Forming Foods:** Avoiding gas-forming foods such as broccoli, cabbage and beans can reduce bloating and gas problems.

Doctor's Advice

If these measures are not enough or if bloating and gas problems become severe, it is important to consult your doctor. Your doctor can assess the situation and recommend more appropriate treatment methods.

Conclusion: Although bloating and gas problems are common during pregnancy, they can be largely controlled with small changes in eating habits and regular physical activity. It is possible to have a comfortable pregnancy by following these tips for a healthy pregnancy.

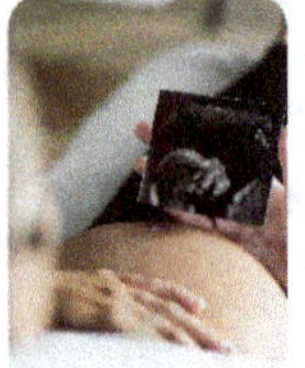
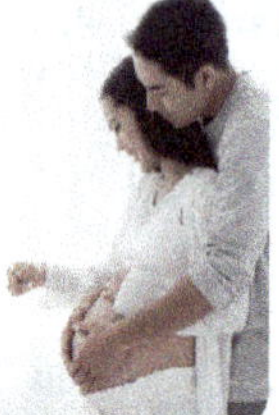
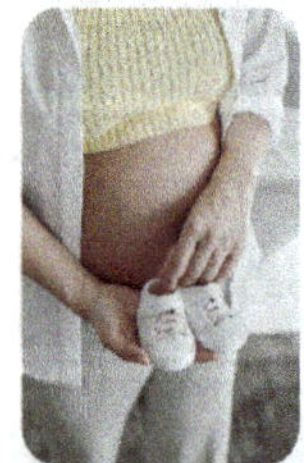
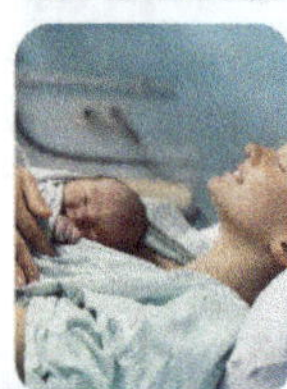

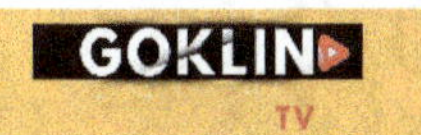

5-WHİCH MEDİCİNES ARE SAFE AND WHİCH ARE DANGEROUS DURİNG PREGNANCY?

It is very important to be careful about the use of medicines during pregnancy. Expectant mothers may want to know which medicines are safe to take to protect the health of their baby. The safety of medicines varies depending on various factors and it is best to seek medical advice in each case. Here is a general guide:

Safe Medicines

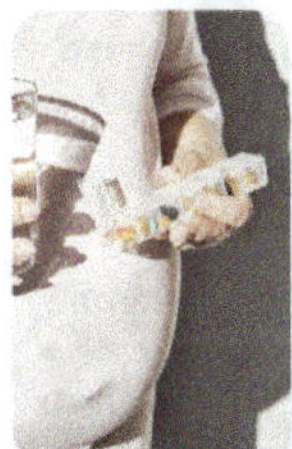

1-Paracetamol (Acetaminophen):
Usage: Paracetamol can be used safely to treat fever and mild to moderate pain.
Caution: It is important to use recommended doses. Overdose should be avoided.
2-Prenatal Vitamins:
Usage: Folic acid, iron, calcium and other vitamins are essential for the healthy development of the baby. Prenatal vitamins should be taken regularly during pregnancy.
3-Some Antacids:
Usage: Heartburn during pregnancy is a common problem and some antacids (for example, calcium carbonate) are considered safe.
Caution: Antacids containing aluminum or magnesium should be avoided.

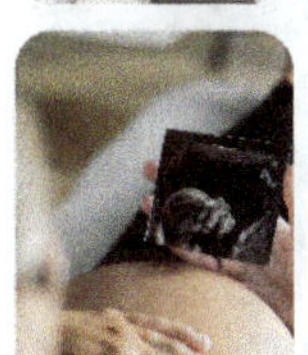

Dangerous Drugs

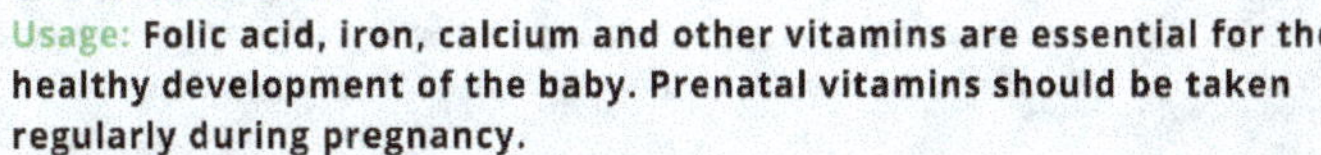

1-Non-Steroidal Anti-Inflammatory Drugs (NSAIDs) (Ibuprofen, Aspirin):
Risks: NSAIDs should not be used during pregnancy, especially in the third trimester. These drugs can cause birth complications and heart problems in the baby.
2-Drugs Containing Retinoids:
Risk: Some medicines used to treat acne (for example, isotretinoin) can cause serious birth defects. Such medicines should be avoided.

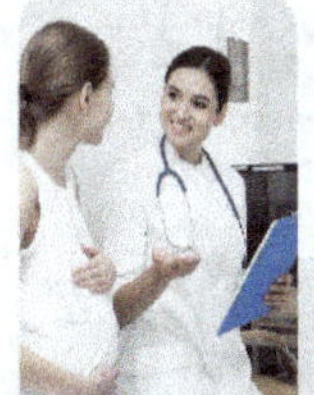

3-Tetracycline Group Antibiotics:
Risk: Tetracyclines can cause permanent staining of the baby's teeth and problems with bone development.

4-ACE Inhibitors and Angiotensin II Receptor Blockers:
Risk: These drugs, which are used to treat high blood pressure, can adversely affect the baby's kidney function and cause low birth weight.

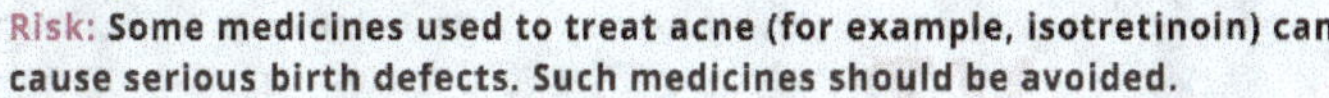

Doctor's Advice and Alternatives
You should always consult your doctor about the use of medication during pregnancy. In some cases, non-drug treatment methods can also be effective. For example, colds and flu can be treated with plenty of fluids, rest and natural remedies.

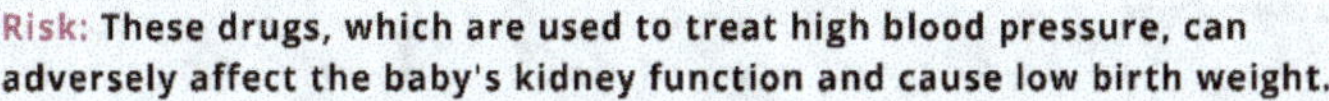

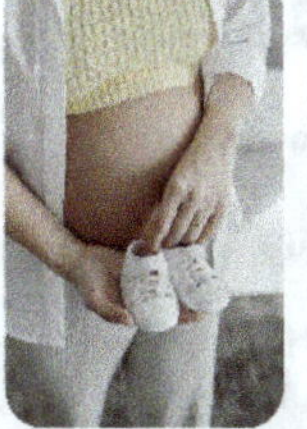

Conclusion: It is vital to be careful when taking medicines during pregnancy and to seek medical advice. By knowing about safe medicines and medicines to avoid, you can protect the health of both mother and baby.

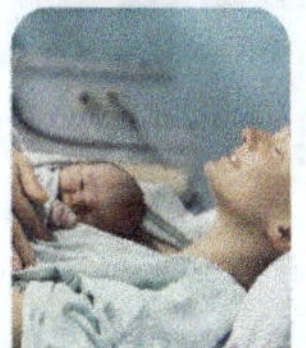

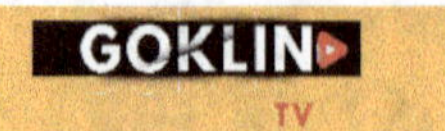

6-WHY DO SKİN CHANGES OCCUR DURİNG PREGNANCY?

Many changes occur in women's bodies during pregnancy. Some of these changes are visible on the skin. The causes of skin changes are hormonal changes, increased blood circulation and changes in body tissues.

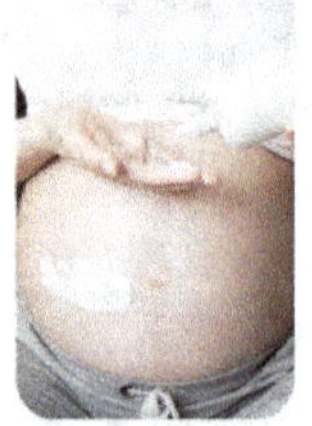

Hormonal changes
During pregnancy, levels of hormones such as estrogen and progesterone increase rapidly. These hormones affect the production and pigmentation of skin cells. The production of a pigment called melanin increases, which leads to darkening of some skin areas. This is known as "melasma" or "pregnancy mask" and usually appears on the face, forehead and cheeks.

Increased Blood Circulation
During pregnancy, blood volume and circulation increase. This can cause redness of the skin and an increase in temperature. In addition, varicose veins can develop, especially in the legs and feet, due to dilated blood vessels. These veins usually return to normal after birth.

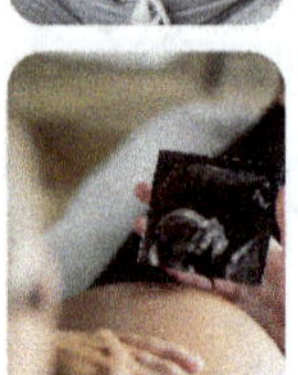

Skin stretching and stretch marks
Skin stretching occurs due to a growing abdomen and weight gain. This stretching can cause small tears in the middle layer of the skin, known as "stretch marks". Stretch marks usually appear on the abdomen, breasts, buttocks and thighs. Initially they may be red or purple, but over time they turn white or silver.

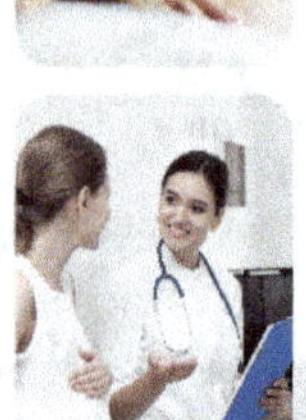
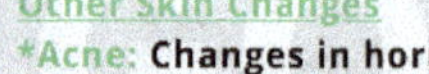
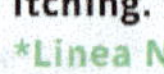

Other Skin Changes
*Acne: Changes in hormone levels can cause acne by increasing oil production in the skin.
*Itching: Stretching and drying of the skin during pregnancy can lead to itching.
*Linea Nigra: The linea nigra, a dark line running vertically down the middle of the abdomen, can become more prominent due to the effect of hormones.

Care and Treatment
Skin changes during pregnancy are usually normal and largely resolve after delivery. However, it is important to pay attention to skin care during this period:

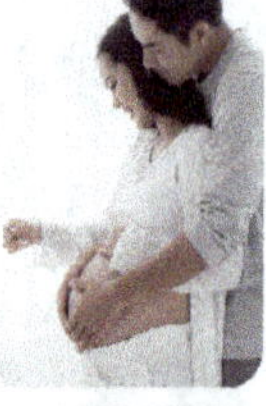

*Use of Moisturizer: Moisturizing the skin can help relieve breakouts and itching.
*Sunscreen: It is beneficial to use sunscreen to reduce pigmentation problems such as melasma.
*Adequate Fluid Consumption: Drinking plenty of water helps keep skin healthy.

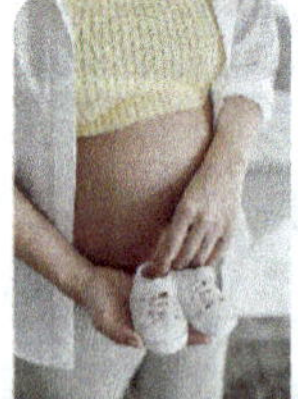

Conclusion: Skin changes during pregnancy are caused by hormonal and physical changes. These changes are usually temporary and return to normal after delivery. It is important to follow proper care and doctor's recommendations for healthy skin.

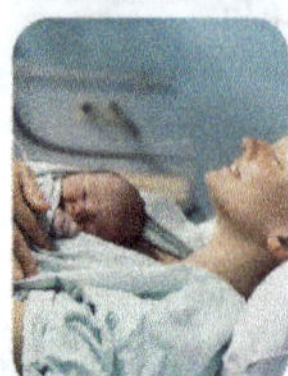

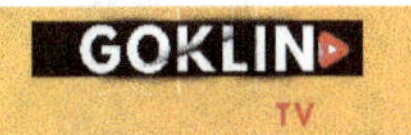

7-HOW TO DEAL WİTH CRAMPS AND PAİN İN PREGNANCY?

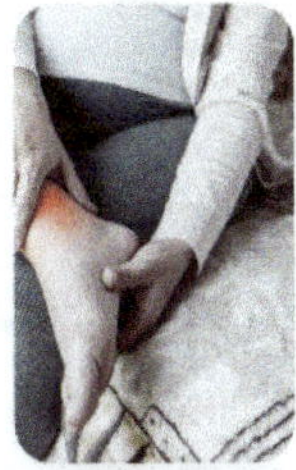

Cramps and aches and pains during pregnancy are common problems that many women face. These conditions are often associated with hormonal changes, an increase in body weight and the growth of the uterus. Fortunately, there are some effective ways to alleviate and manage these discomforts.

Cramps in Pregnancy

Cramps are sudden muscle spasms, usually felt in the legs and feet. During pregnancy, cramps can occur frequently, especially at night.

Coping Methods:

1- Stretching Exercises:

To stretch your leg muscles before going to bed, you can do 2-3 sets of stretching exercises for each leg by pulling your fingertips up and holding them for a few seconds.

2- Adequate Fluid Consumption:

Drinking at least 8-10 glasses (2-2.5 liters) of water throughout the day ensures hydration of the muscles and prevents cramps.

3-Magnesium Supplement:

Consume magnesium-rich foods such as spinach, almonds, cashews. With the recommendation of your doctor, 350-400 mg of magnesium supplements can be taken daily.

4-Massage and Hot Compress:

Relax the muscles by lightly massaging the cramped area and applying a hot water bottle.

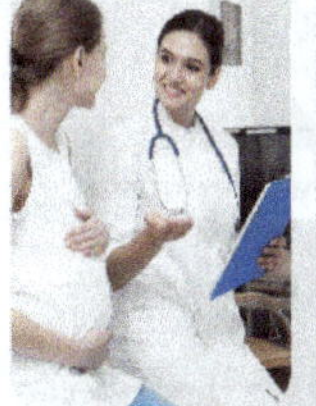

Pain in Pregnancy

Pain is common during pregnancy, especially in the back, lower back and buttocks. These pains are caused by the growth of the uterus, hormonal changes and a change in the body's center of gravity.

Coping Methods:

1-Correct Posture:

When sitting, your feet should be flat on the floor, your back should be straight and you should use a small pillow to support your lower back if necessary.

When standing, pull your shoulders back and stand up straight. Avoid standing for long periods of time.

2-Supportive Shoes:

Choose shoes with a heel height of 2-4 cm that provide good support.

3-Exercise:

-20-30 minutes of light brisk walking a day strengthens muscles and increases flexibility.

-Swimming 2-3 times a week for 30 minutes relieves back and lower back pain.

-Practicing yoga 2-3 times a week for 20-30 minutes stretches muscles and promotes relaxation.

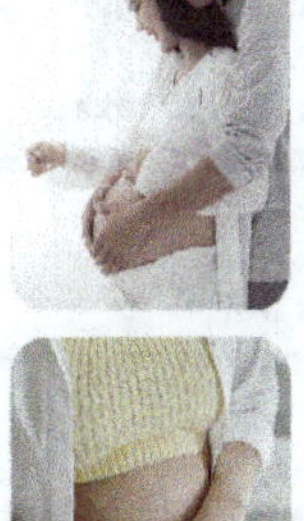

4-Hot and Cold Therapy:

Apply a hot water bottle or cold compress for 15-20 minutes 2-3 times a day for back and lower back pain.

5-Support pillows:

When sleeping on your side, sleep with support pillows between your legs and on your back. Maintain the alignment of your body.

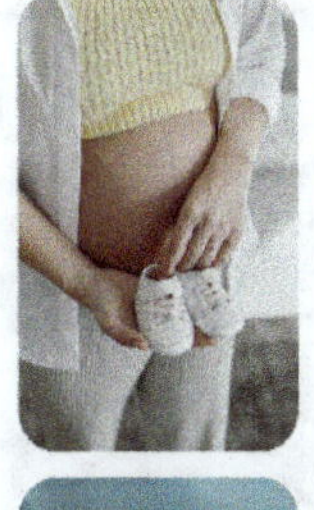

Doctor's Advice

If the cramps and pain are severe or persistent, you should consult your doctor. Your doctor will assess the situation and give you the most appropriate treatment and advice.

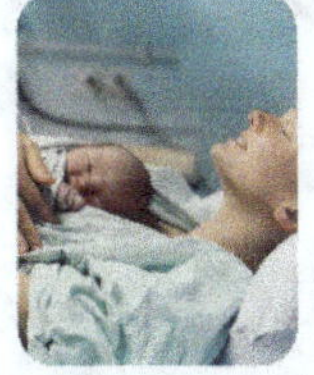

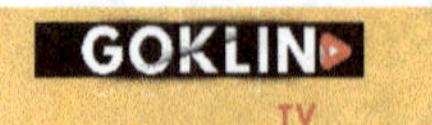

8-FLİGHT TRAVEL DURİNG PREGNANCY: IS IT SAFE?

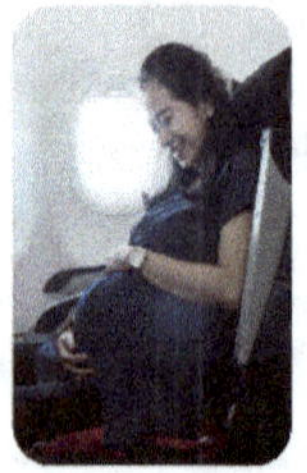

Traveling by plane during pregnancy is generally safe, but in some cases it is necessary to be careful. Expectant mothers should pay attention to a few important points when making travel plans during pregnancy.

1. Period of Pregnancy:

- **First trimester (first 12 weeks):** During this period, it is recommended to avoid long trips as the risk of miscarriage is higher. Also, pregnancy symptoms such as nausea and fatigue may be more intense during this period.
- **Second trimester (13-28 weeks):** This is the best period for traveling during pregnancy. Energy levels are usually higher and the risk of miscarriage is reduced. Most doctors allow pregnant women to fly during this period.
- **Third trimester (29 weeks and beyond):** During this period, there may be travel restrictions due to the risk of premature birth. Most airlines do not allow pregnant women to fly after 36 weeks and usually require a doctor's note after 28 weeks.

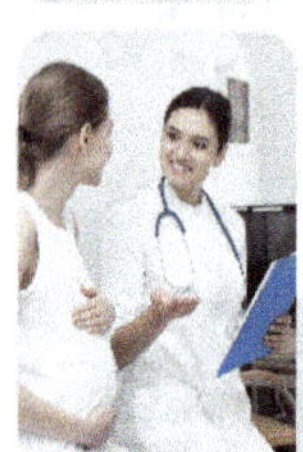

2. Flight Duration and Quantity:

- **Short-haul flights (1-2 hours):** Generally safe and can be done comfortably during pregnancy.
- **Medium distance flights (3-5 hours):** Still safe, but it is recommended to get up and take short walks every hour or so to avoid long periods of inactivity.
- **Long-haul flights (6 hours or more):** On such flights, it is important to move frequently and drink plenty of water to improve blood circulation. Also, wearing compression stockings that cover the legs can reduce the risk of deep vein thrombosis.

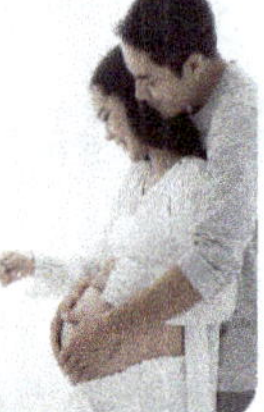

3. Travel Preparations and Precautions:

- **Consultation with the Doctor:** Always consult your doctor before flying and confirm that air travel is safe for you.
- **Movement and Stretching:** During long flights, it is important to take a walk in the aisle every hour, stretch the legs and do exercises to improve blood circulation.
- **Drink plenty of water:** The dry air inside the airplane can dehydrate the body. Therefore, it is very important to drink plenty of water.
- **Comfortable Clothing:** Wearing comfortable, loose clothing and supportive shoes will increase your comfort.

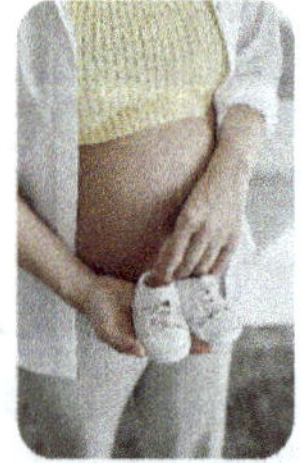

Conclusion: Traveling by plane during pregnancy is generally safe, but it is important to always talk to your doctor to get the best advice for your individual situation.

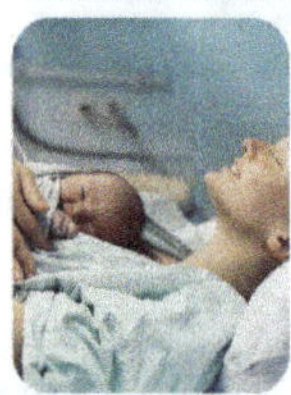

9-DİSEASES İN THE BABY DURİNG PREGNANCY: WHAT ARE THEY AND HOW TO MANAGE THEM?

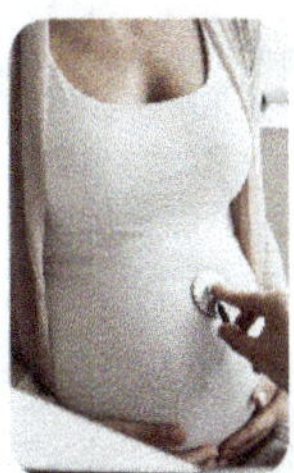

The health of the baby during pregnancy is one of the most important issues for expectant mothers. Some prenatal health problems can occur in the baby and early diagnosis and management of these conditions is very important for the baby to be born healthy. Here are some of the diseases that can occur in the baby during pregnancy and information about the management of these diseases:

1. Congenital Anomalies (Birth Defects):

- **Definition:** Structural or functional abnormalities that occur in the baby before birth. There are various types such as heart defects, neural tube defects (spina bifida) and cleft lip and palate.

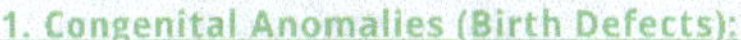

- **Diagnosis:** Anomalies are usually detected by routine ultrasound scans. A detailed ultrasound in the second trimester, especially between 18 and 22 weeks, can detect most birth defects. In addition, fetal echocardiography, magnetic resonance imaging (MRI) or genetic testing may be needed in some cases.

2. Genetic Diseases:

- **Definition:** Health problems caused by genetic mutations or inherited diseases in the baby. Diseases such as Down syndrome, cystic fibrosis, sickle cell anemia, Tay-Sachs disease and thalassemia fall into this group.
- **Diagnosis:** Genetic diseases are diagnosed through various prenatal tests.

These include

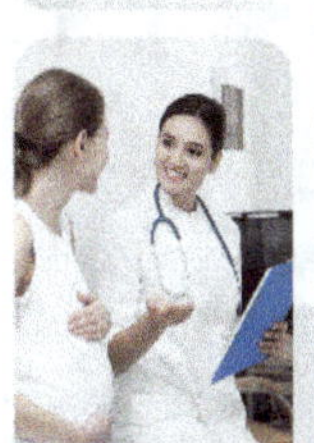

- **Amniocentesis:** Taking a sample of amniotic fluid and analyzing it. It is usually performed between weeks 15 and 20 and is used to detect chromosomal abnormalities and some genetic diseases.
- **Chorionic Villus Biopsy (CVS):** Genetic analysis of a small tissue sample from the placenta. It can be performed between weeks 10-13 and is used to detect chromosomal abnormalities and some genetic diseases.
- **Non-invasive Prenatal Tests (NIPT):** An analysis of the baby's DNA using a sample of the mother's blood. These tests are particularly effective in detecting chromosomal abnormalities such as Down syndrome, Edwards syndrome and Patau syndrome.
- **Fetal DNA Analysis:** This can be done with samples taken from the womb or placenta. These analyses can detect the presence of certain genetic mutations or diseases.

3. Fetal Growth Retardation (IUGR):

- **Definition:** Intrauterine growth retardation (IUGR) occurs when the baby grows more slowly than expected during pregnancy.
- **Diagnosis:** IUGR is detected by monitoring the baby's growth rate with regular ultrasound scans. Doppler ultrasound can help identify the presence of IUGR by examining the baby's blood flow. The mother's blood pressure and urine tests can also be used to assess IUGR.

4. Prenatal Infections:

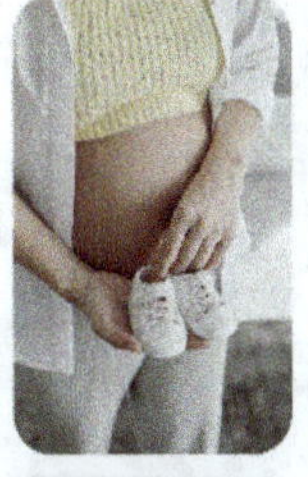

- **Definition:** If the expectant mother gets infections during pregnancy, these infections can be passed on to the baby. Infections such as toxoplasmosis, CMV and Zika virus fall into this group.
- **Diagnosis:** Prenatal infections can be detected by blood tests and ultrasound scans. The presence of specific antibodies in the mother's blood can indicate the presence of infection.

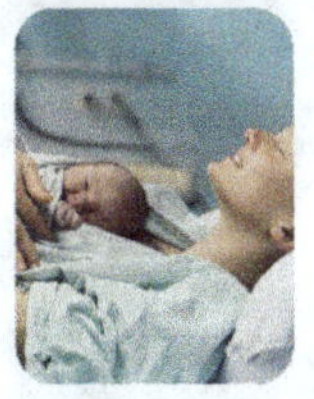

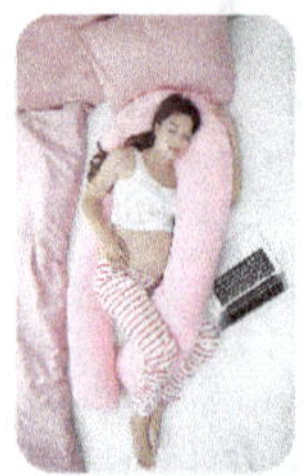

Maintaining sleep patterns during pregnancy is very important for the health of both the expectant mother and the baby. Hormonal changes, physical ailments and stress during pregnancy can negatively affect your sleep patterns. Here are some scientific recommendations for maintaining sleep patterns:

1. Sleep Position:

- **Recommendation:** During the second and third trimesters of pregnancy, it is best to sleep on your left side. This position increases blood flow and the delivery of nutrients to the placenta.
- **Detail:** You can make yourself more comfortable by placing a pillow between your legs and on your back. This can reduce lower back and hip pain.

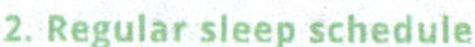

2. Regular sleep schedule:

- **Recommendation:** Establish a regular sleep schedule by going to bed and getting up at the same time every day.
- **Detail:** Try to get 7-9 hours of sleep. Create a relaxing routine (such as taking a hot shower or reading a book) before going to sleep.

3. Suitable sleep environment:

- **Suggestion:** Keep your bedroom cool, dark and quiet. Use a comfortable mattress and pillows.
- **Detail:** Stop using electronic devices (phone, tablet, TV) at least one hour before bedtime. The blue light emitted by these devices can suppress the hormone melatonin, making it difficult to fall asleep.

4. Fluid Consumption and Nutrition:

- **Recommendation:** Avoid heavy meals and caffeinated drinks before bedtime. Avoid drinking too much fluid 1-2 hours before bedtime.
- **Detail:** A light snack (such as a handful of almonds or a glass of milk) can help prevent feelings of hunger during the night.

5. Exercise:

- **Recommendation:** Regular light exercise can improve the quality of your sleep. However, avoid intense exercise just before going to sleep.
- **Detail:** Walking for at least 30 minutes a day can help you fall asleep easier.

By taking these tips into account, you can improve your physical well-being and get a better quality of sleep during pregnancy. Regular sleep will help you feel more energized and healthy throughout your pregnancy.

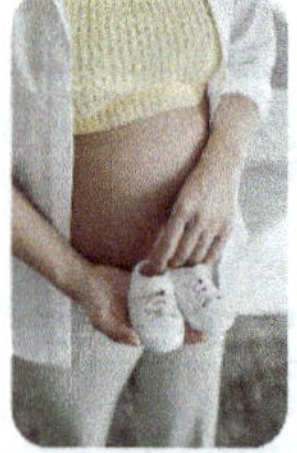

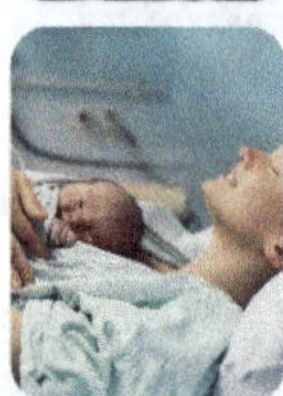

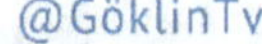

11-WHEN ARE ULTRASOUND AND OTHER SCANS PERFORMED DURING PREGNANCY?

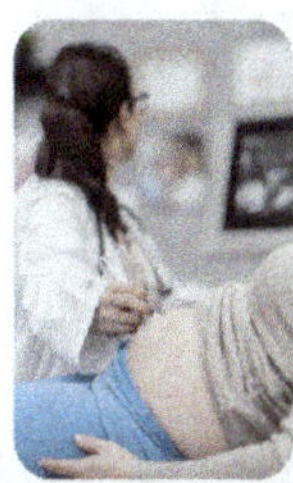

Ultrasounds and other scans during pregnancy are vital for monitoring the health of mother and baby and detecting potential problems early. These scans can detect serious health problems such as Down syndrome, spina bifida, heart defects and other genetic and structural anomalies. Early detection allows appropriate treatment and intervention plans to be put in place, ensuring a healthy pregnancy for both mother and baby. In addition, these screenings help the expectant mother to relax psychologically and better prepare for the birth process.

1st Trimester: First Trimester Screenings (0-13 weeks)

- **First Ultrasound:** It is done between 6-9 weeks of pregnancy. This ultrasound is used to confirm the pregnancy, see the gestational sac and embryo, and detect the heartbeat. It also checks the baby's location (inside or outside the uterus).
- **Dual Screening Test:** It is done between 11-14 weeks. This test uses a combination of ultrasound and blood tests to assess the risk of Down syndrome and other genetic disorders. The nuchal translucency of the baby is measured and some hormone levels in the mother's blood are analyzed.

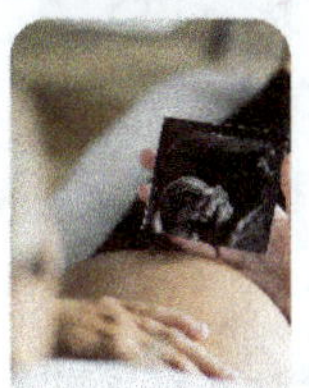

2nd Trimester: Second Trimester Scans (14-26 weeks)

- **Detailed Ultrasound (Anomaly Screening):** It is performed between 18-22 weeks. This ultrasound examines the baby's anatomy in detail, assessing organ development, brain, heart, kidneys and other structures. It also checks the position of the placenta and the amount of amniotic fluid.
- **Triple or Quadruple Screening Test:** This is done between weeks 15 and 20. These blood tests assess the baby's risk for neural tube defects such as spina bifida and other genetic disorders.

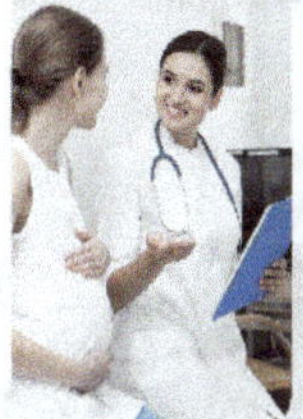

3rd Trimester: Third Trimester Scans (27-40 weeks)

- **Growth Ultrasound:** It is performed between 28-32 weeks. This ultrasound is used to assess the baby's growth rate and weight estimation, and to check the amount of amniotic fluid.
- **Non-Stress Test (NST):** After 32 weeks, especially in high-risk pregnancies, it is used to monitor the baby's heartbeat and movements.
- **Biophysical Profile:** This test, performed after 32 weeks, uses a combination of ultrasound and NST to assess the baby's health.

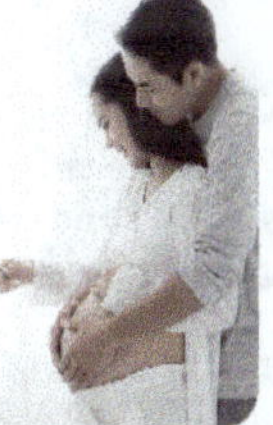

These scans are carried out to ensure a healthy pregnancy for the baby and the mother. Every pregnancy is different and doctors may recommend additional tests or different timing depending on the individual needs of the expectant mother. It is therefore important to follow regular check-ups and follow the advice of your doctor.

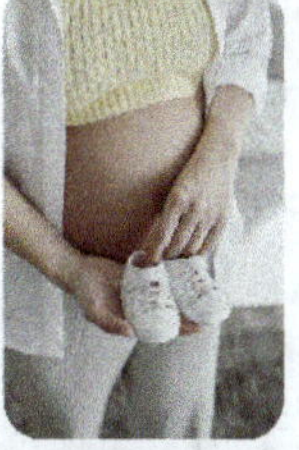

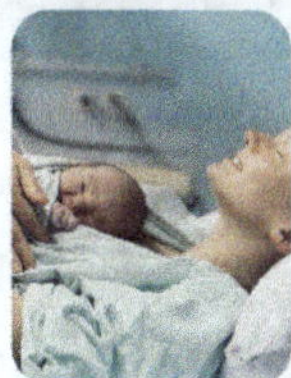

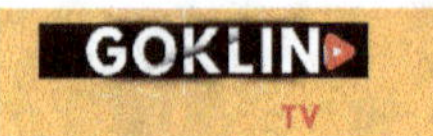

12-WHEN CAN I FEEL THE BABY'S MOVEMENTS DURING PREGNANCY?

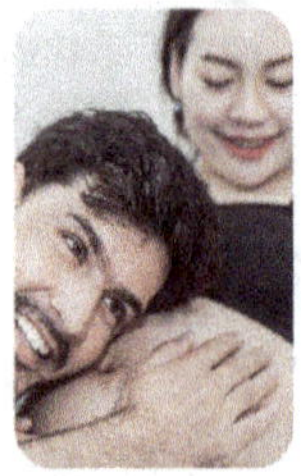

One of the most eagerly awaited moments during pregnancy is feeling the baby's movements. Feeling the baby's first movements strengthens the bond between the expectant mother and her baby and has great significance as a sign of the progress of the pregnancy. These movements are usually felt between the 16th and 25th week of pregnancy.

First movements (quickening)
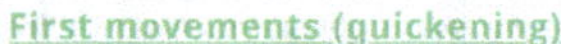
Women in their first pregnancy usually start to feel the baby's movements between 18 and 25 weeks. In second or subsequent pregnancies, expectant mothers may feel them earlier, usually around 16 weeks. This is because they know what the movements felt like in previous pregnancies and are more familiar with the sensation.

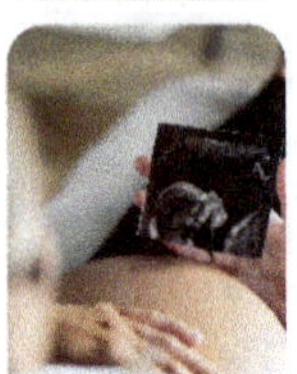

How to feel the baby's movements?
At first, the baby's movements can be very light and vague. Expectant mothers often describe them as "butterfly fluttering" or "gas bubbles". Over time, as the baby gets bigger and stronger, these movements become more pronounced and stronger. After 24 weeks, the baby may start kicking and turning and the expectant mother can feel these movements more clearly.

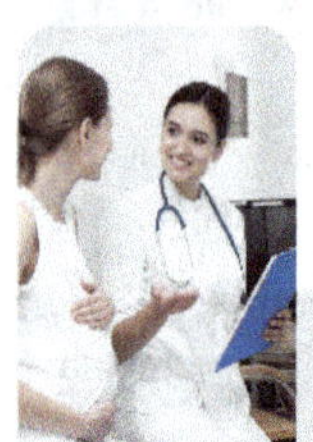

Regularity of Movements
Babies move regularly in the womb and usually have a set pattern of movement. Babies have periods of sleeping and waking and the intensity of their movements can change during these periods. Expectant mothers may feel their baby's movements more intensely at certain times of the day. Especially when the expectant mother is resting or after eating, the baby's movements may be more pronounced.

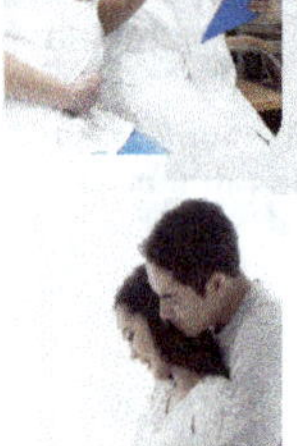

Monitoring Movements
Later in pregnancy, doctors may ask expectant mothers to keep track of the baby's movements and note how many movements they feel over a period of time. This is an important way to check the baby's health and well-being. If a sudden decrease or change in baby movements is noticed, a doctor should be consulted immediately.

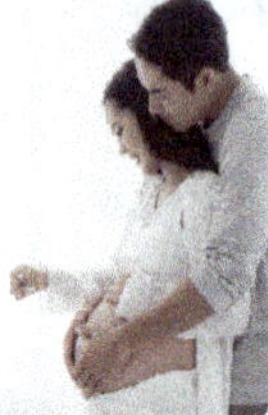

Not Feeling Movements
Feeling the baby's movements may not occur at the same time for every expectant mother. Factors such as the position of the baby, the location of the placenta and the mother's weight can affect the timing of the movements. This can be a concern for first-time moms, but every pregnancy is different and the baby's health is regularly monitored during check-ups.

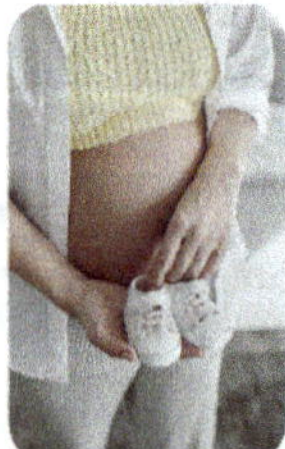

Feeling the baby's movements during pregnancy is a way for the expectant mother to bond with her baby, as well as an indication that the baby is growing healthily. It is therefore important to pay attention to the information provided by the doctor about when and how movements are felt.

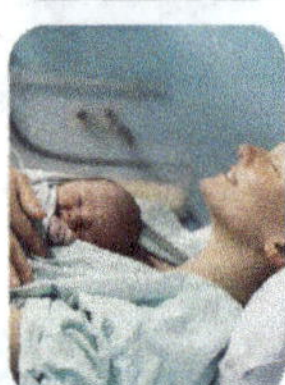

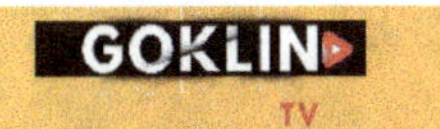

13-HOW TO PREVENT ANEMİA AND IRON DEFİCİENCY İN PREGNANCY?

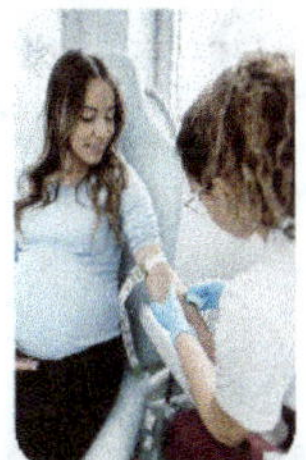

Anemia and iron deficiency during pregnancy are common problems that expectant mothers may face. Anemia is a condition in which there are not enough red blood cells in the blood, which are needed to carry oxygen. Iron deficiency anemia, on the other hand, is caused by a deficiency of the mineral iron and is more common during pregnancy due to the increased need for iron. Anemia can present with symptoms such as fatigue, weakness, dizziness and pale skin. However, it is possible to prevent this condition with appropriate precautions.

1.Consume iron-rich foods

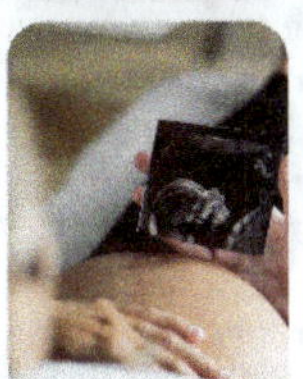

To prevent iron deficiency, it is important to include iron-rich foods in your diet. Animal sources such as red meat, chicken, fish, liver are the best sources of iron. Also, green leafy vegetables (spinach, chard), legumes (lentils, chickpeas), dried fruits (raisins, apricots) and whole grains are good sources of plant iron.

2.Increase Iron Absorption with Vitamin C

Vitamin C helps the body absorb iron better. Therefore, it is beneficial to consume foods containing vitamin C along with iron-rich foods. Foods such as oranges, tangerines, strawberries, kiwi, broccoli and peppers are rich in vitamin C.

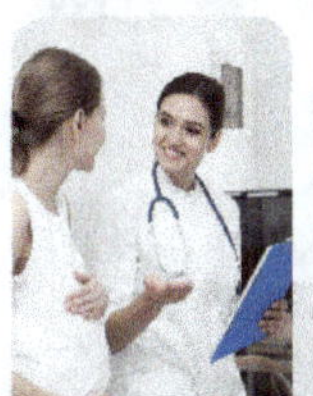
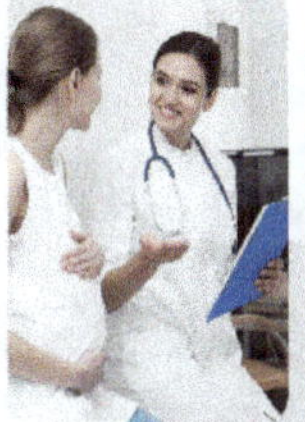

3.Limit Tea and Coffee Consumption

Drinks such as tea and coffee contain substances that reduce iron absorption. Therefore, limiting or completely avoiding the consumption of these drinks with meals can improve iron absorption. It is better to consume these drinks at least one hour before or after meals.

4.Use Iron Supplements

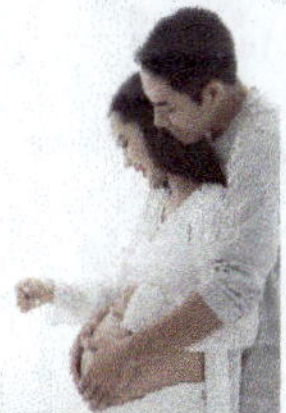

Your doctor will monitor your iron levels and may prescribe iron supplements as needed. It is important to take iron supplements in the dose and duration recommended by your doctor, especially if you have been diagnosed with iron deficiency anemia. Supplements are usually recommended during the second and third trimesters of pregnancy.

5.Have regular blood tests

It is important to have regular blood tests during pregnancy to monitor your iron levels. These tests help to detect anemia or iron deficiency early and ensure that the necessary measures are taken in time.

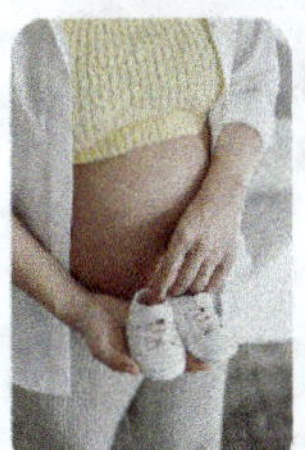

Preventing anemia and iron deficiency during pregnancy is critical for the health of both the expectant mother and the baby. A balanced and nutritious diet, iron absorption supported by vitamin C, control of tea and coffee consumption and the use of iron supplements when necessary will be effective in preventing these problems. It is also important to monitor your health with regular medical check-ups and blood tests. With these measures, you can have a healthy pregnancy and give your baby the best start.

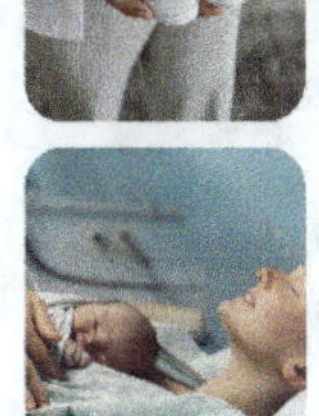

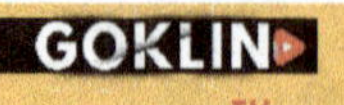

14-HOW TO PREPARE A BİRTH PLAN DURİNG PREGNANCY?

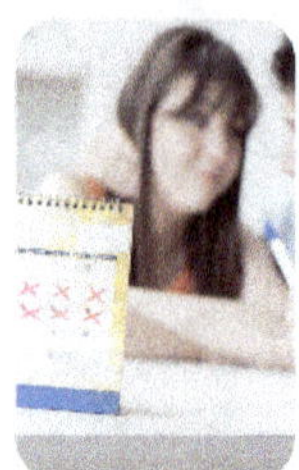

Preparing a birth plan during pregnancy helps both the expectant mother and the health care team to set expectations and preferences for the birth as the due date approaches. A birth plan is a written document that clearly states what you want to happen and what you want to avoid during the birth process.

Here is the step-by-step process of preparing a birth plan;

1. Do Research

Before starting to prepare a birth plan, it is important to learn about the birth process. Learn about the different methods of delivery (normal delivery, caesarean section, water birth), pain management options (epidural, drug-free delivery), techniques that can be used during labor (breathing techniques, changing positions) and postnatal care. This information will help you make more informed choices.

2. Talk to your health team

Talk to your doctor and your birth team before making your birth plan. Find out about the hospital's birth policies, services and facilities. Some hospitals may not accept certain practices, so it is important to align your plan with your healthcare team.

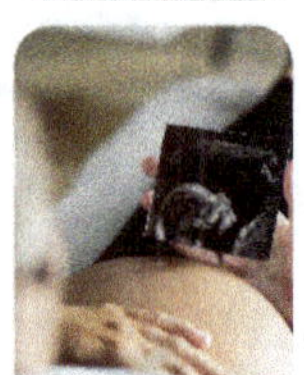

3. Identify your preferences

Here are some basic things that should be included in your birth plan;

- **Birth Environment:** If you prefer to give birth in a hospital, birth center or at home, indicate this. You can also write down how you would like the room to be (lighting, music, etc.).
- **Pain Management:** Indicate pain management options such as pain medication or epidural anesthesia. If you prefer natural methods, indicate this as well.
- **Birth Positions:** Write down which birth positions you prefer. You can choose from standing, squatting, lying on your side, etc.
- **People you want to be with you during labor:** Indicate if you would like people such as your partner, a family member or a doula to be with you during labor.

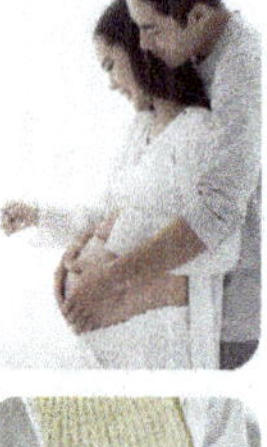

- **Postpartum Care:** If you would prefer to be able to hold your baby immediately after birth, to start breastfeeding immediately or to be left alone for a certain period of time, write down your wishes.
-

4. Be Flexible

It is important to leave wiggle room in your birth plan. Birth may not go as planned due to unforeseen circumstances. Be open to suggestions from your health care team and be ready to adapt your plan as needed.

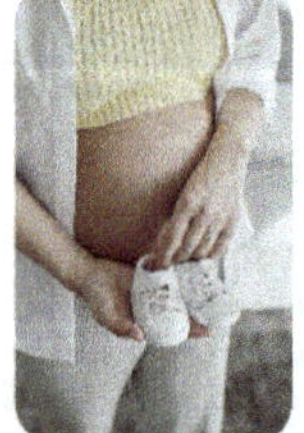

5. Put your birth plan in writing

Prepare your birth plan in writing and, if possible, summarize it in no more than one page. Use clear and understandable language and express your preferences clearly. Share your plan with your doctor and birth team so that they are aware of your plan.

A birth plan can make the birth process more manageable and less stressful. Identifying your own preferences is key to making your birth experience personal and satisfying. Remember, this is your birth and you have the right to express your preferences.

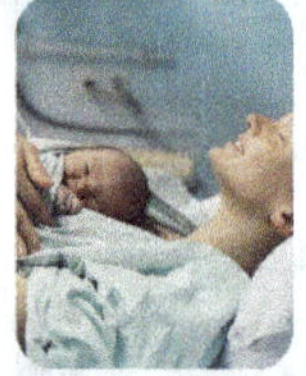

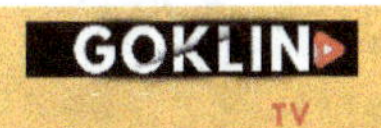

15-IS SEXUAL INTERCOURSE SAFE DURING PREGNANCY?

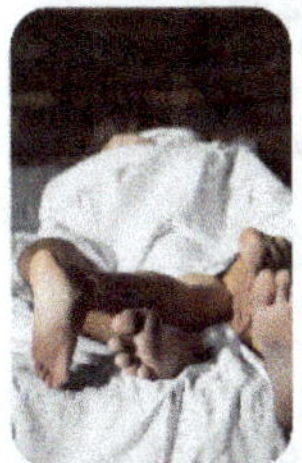

Sexual intercourse during pregnancy is safe in most cases and can be part of a healthy relationship for couples. One of the most common concerns about sex during pregnancy is the risk of harming the baby. However, unless there are pregnancy complications, sexual intercourse does not harm the baby and does not threaten the health of the expectant mother.

1. Protecting the baby

Inside the uterus, your baby is protected by the amniotic sac and strong uterine muscles. This protective structure prevents the baby from being harmed during sexual intercourse. In addition, the mucus plug in the cervix prevents infections from entering the uterus.

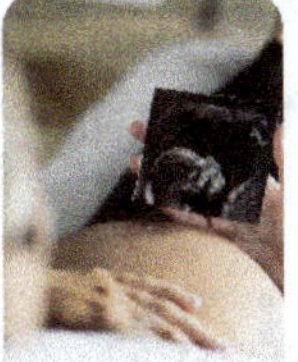

2. Benefits of sexual intercourse

Sexual intercourse can strengthen the emotional bond between couples during pregnancy and reduce stress levels. Orgasm can help the expectant mother feel better by increasing the release of endorphins. In addition, intercourse can increase blood circulation and strengthen the pelvic muscles.

3.Position Selection

As pregnancy progresses, some sexual positions can be uncomfortable. In this case, it is important to try positions that are comfortable for the expectant mother. For example, sexual intercourse lying side by side or positions where the woman is on top can be more comfortable during pregnancy. Pressure on the abdomen should be avoided.

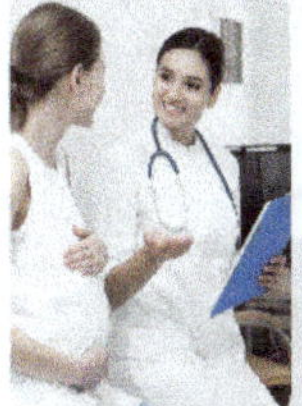
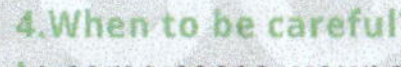

4.When to be careful?

In some cases, your doctor may advise you to limit or completely avoid sexual intercourse. These situations include:
  • Risk of miscarriage or a history of miscarriage
  • Risk of preterm labor or threat of preterm labor
  • Placenta previa (placenta covering the cervix)
  • Vaginal bleeding or abnormal discharge
  • Leakage or rupture of amniotic fluid
  • Multiple pregnancy (such as twins, triplets)
In such cases, it is important to follow your doctor's advice and be careful about sexual intercourse.

5. Communication with the partner

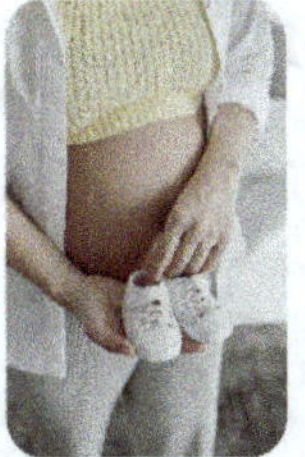

It is important to talk openly and honestly with your partner about sex. Share your thoughts and feelings so that both of you feel comfortable and safe. If you have concerns about sex during pregnancy, do not hesitate to discuss them with your doctor.

Conclusion: Sexual intercourse during pregnancy is generally safe and can be part of a healthy relationship between couples. However, it is important to follow your doctor's advice if there are any complications or risks. Communication and careful behavior is always the best approach for a healthy pregnancy.

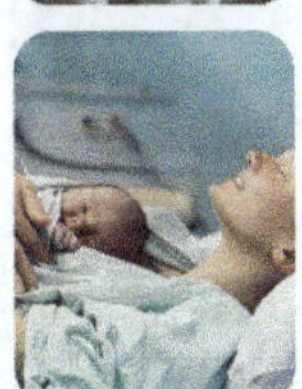

16-WHICH VACCINATIONS SHOULD BE GIVEN DURING PREGNANCY?

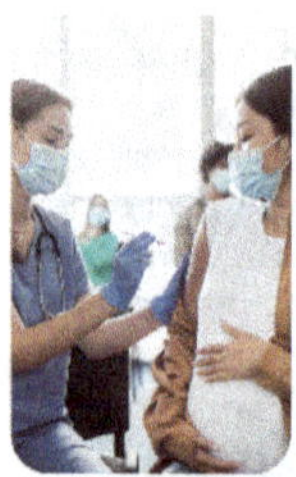

Some vaccines are recommended to protect the health of the expectant mother and baby during pregnancy. These vaccines protect the expectant mother from infections and protect the baby in the postnatal period. Here are the vaccines recommended during pregnancy:

1. Flu Vaccine

Influenza can lead to serious complications during pregnancy and threaten the health of both the expectant mother and the baby. Therefore, the flu vaccine is one of the most important vaccinations recommended during pregnancy. The flu vaccine not only protects the expectant mother from the flu, but also reduces the risk of the baby getting the flu in the first few months after birth. The flu vaccine can be given safely at any time during pregnancy.

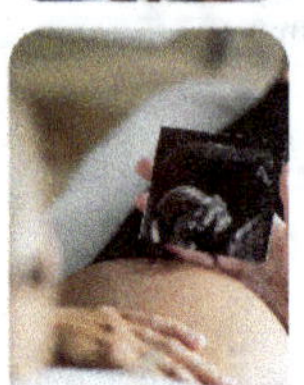

2.Tdap Vaccine (Tetanus, Diphtheria and Pertussis)

The Tdap vaccine protects against tetanus, diphtheria and whooping cough. Whooping cough (pertussis) in particular can be very dangerous for babies and can cause serious breathing problems. For this reason, the Tdap vaccine is recommended between 27-36 weeks of pregnancy. This vaccine boosts the mother's immunity and provides passive immunity to the baby after birth.

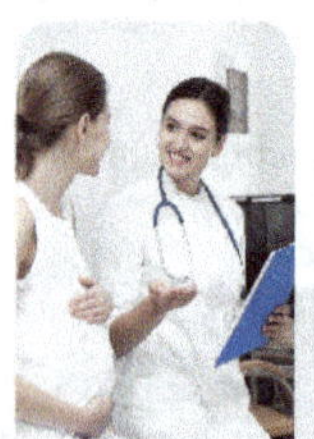

3.Hepatitis B Vaccine

Hepatitis B is a serious infection that can lead to liver damage. Mothers who have hepatitis B during pregnancy can pass the virus to their babies during childbirth. If the expectant mother does not have hepatitis B, the hepatitis B vaccine may be recommended. The vaccine can be given safely at any time during pregnancy.

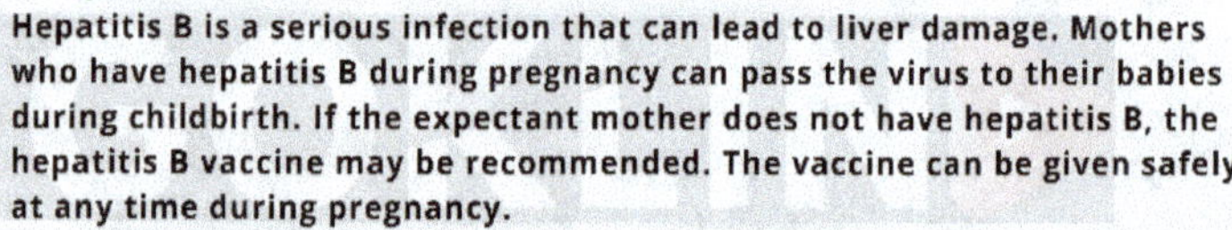

Things to Consider Before Vaccination:

- **Talk to Your Doctor:** Talk to your doctor about which vaccines should be given during pregnancy. Determine the most appropriate vaccination schedule based on your personal health history and the condition of your pregnancy.
- **Vaccine Schedule:** The timing of planned vaccinations should be arranged to best protect the health of the mother and baby.
- **Side Effects:** Side effects of vaccines are usually mild and temporary. They may include mild fever, muscle pain and tenderness at the injection site. Severe side effects are rare, but contact your doctor if you have any concerns.

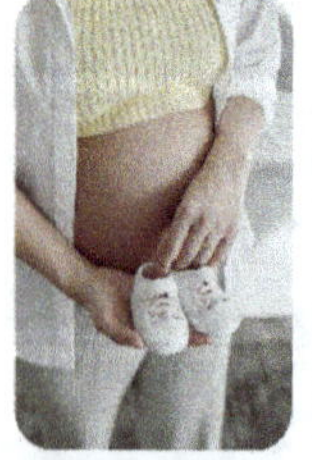

Vaccinations during pregnancy play an important role in protecting the health of the expectant mother and baby. Regular medical check-ups and the recommended vaccinations are essential for a healthy pregnancy and delivery. Vaccinations provide protection against infections and ensure the health of both mother and baby.

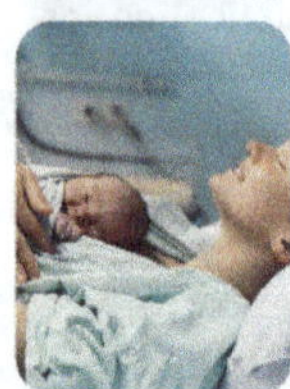

17-WHAT İS GESTATİONAL DİABETES İN PREGNANCY AND HOW İS İT MANAGED?

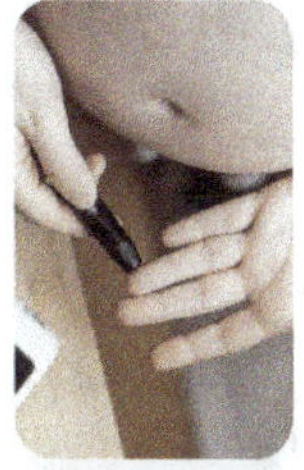

WHAT İS GESTATİONAL DİABETES?

Gestational diabetes is a type of diabetes that occurs during pregnancy and usually disappears when the pregnancy ends. The condition occurs when the body is unable to produce enough insulin or to use it effectively, resulting in blood sugar levels above normal. Gestational diabetes can carry some health risks for both mother and baby. Therefore, proper management and treatment methods are very important.

How to Manage Gestational Diabetes?

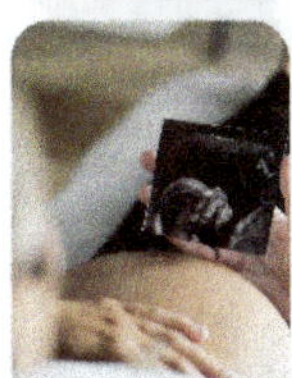

1-Regular Blood Sugar Control: Regularly checking blood glucose levels during pregnancy is a key step in managing gestational diabetes. Your doctor will determine how often you should measure blood glucose and set target blood glucose levels.

2-Healthy Nutrition: One of the most effective ways to manage gestational diabetes is to follow a healthy and balanced diet. Your eating plan should include complex carbohydrates, fiber, protein and healthy fats. Avoid foods that raise blood sugar quickly, such as white bread, sugary foods and processed foods. Consuming your meals at regular intervals and in small portions helps to keep blood sugar levels in balance.

3-Regular Exercise: Exercise plays an important role in the management of gestational diabetes. Regular physical activity can help lower blood sugar and increase the effect of insulin. Light to moderate exercise, especially walking and swimming, is safe and beneficial during pregnancy. It is important to consult your doctor before starting your exercise program.

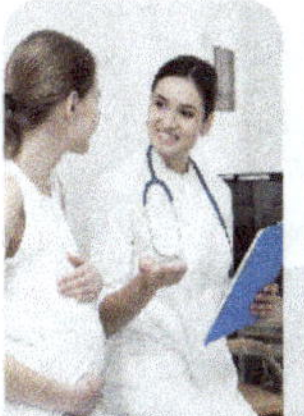

4-Insulin Therapy: When diet and exercise are insufficient to control blood sugar levels, your doctor may recommend insulin therapy. Insulin helps the body regulate blood sugar and protects the baby's health. Your doctor will guide you on how to give insulin injections.

5-Regular Doctor Check-ups: It is very important to go for regular doctor check-ups during the gestational diabetes management process. Your doctor will monitor your blood glucose levels, perform the necessary tests and assess your health. Additional tests, such as ultrasound, may also be performed to prevent potential complications of gestational diabetes.

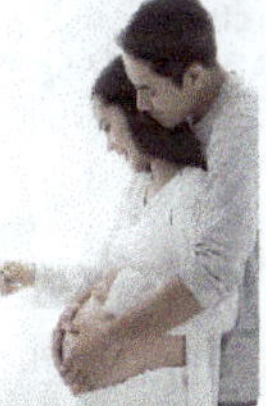

Risks and Precautions: Gestational diabetes can carry risks such as birth complications, high birth weight and the development of postpartum diabetes. Therefore, it is vital to follow your doctor's recommendations and make the necessary lifestyle changes when you are diagnosed with gestational diabetes. A healthy diet, regular exercise and regular medical check-ups can help manage gestational diabetes and ensure a healthy pregnancy for both mother and baby.

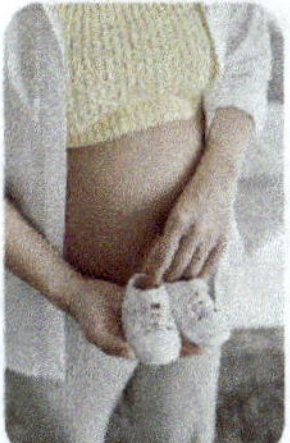

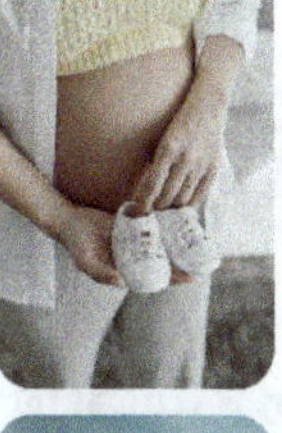

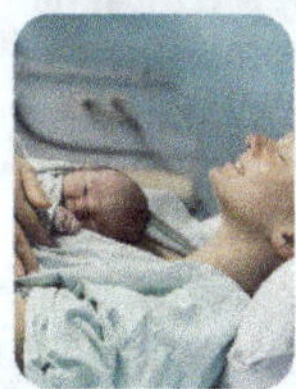

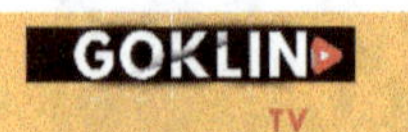

18-HOW TO CONTROL HİGH BLOOD PRESSURE İN PREGNANCY?

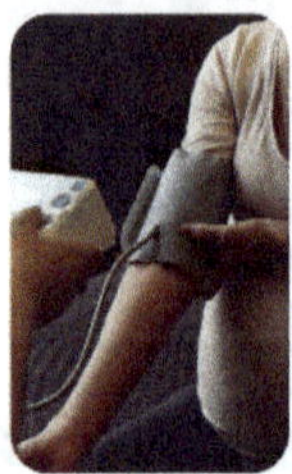

High blood pressure (hypertension) during pregnancy is an important condition that can affect the health of the expectant mother and the baby. High blood pressure can lead to serious complications such as pre-eclampsia. Therefore, it is very important to control and manage blood pressure during pregnancy. Here are some ways to control high blood pressure during pregnancy:

1. Regular Doctor Check-ups: Regular visits to the doctor during pregnancy are critical to closely monitor blood pressure. Your doctor will measure your blood pressure levels regularly and take the necessary measures if any abnormalities are detected. Urine tests and blood tests may also be done to monitor for signs of pre-eclampsia.

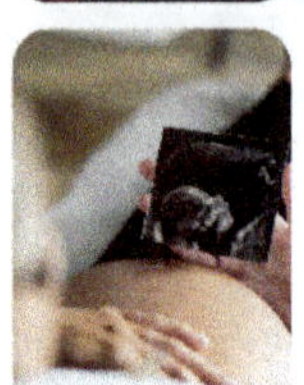

2. Healthy Diet: A balanced and healthy diet plays an important role in keeping blood pressure under control. Eating a diet that includes fresh fruits and vegetables, whole grains, lean proteins and healthy fats can help stabilize your blood pressure. Reducing salt consumption is also effective in controlling blood pressure, as excessive salt consumption can cause blood pressure to rise.

3. Regular Exercise: Regular exercise can help lower blood pressure. Light to moderate exercise is safe and recommended during pregnancy. Activities such as walking, swimming and prenatal yoga keep blood pressure under control and promote overall health. Before starting your exercise program, it is important to talk to your doctor to determine which exercises are suitable for you.

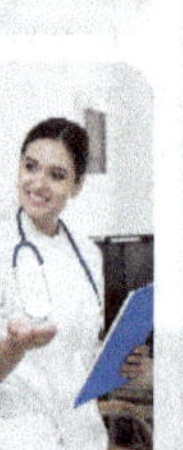
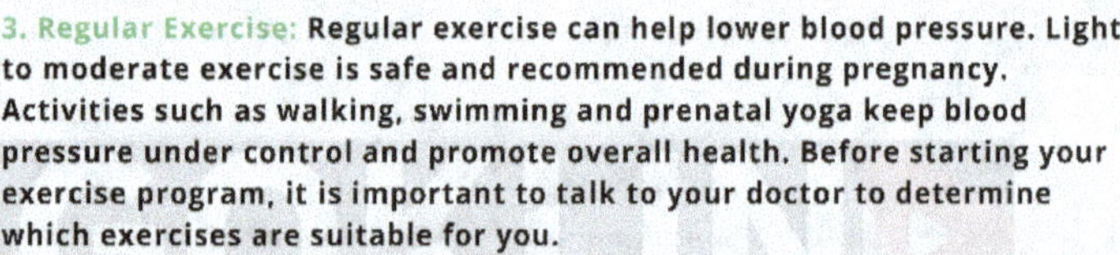

4. Stress Management: Stress can contribute to high blood pressure. Methods such as relaxation techniques, deep breathing exercises and meditation can be used to reduce stress during pregnancy. Also, getting enough sleep and engaging in relaxing activities can help lower your stress levels.

5. Medication: In some cases, your doctor may recommend medication to control high blood pressure. Blood pressure medications used during pregnancy are selected from those that are safe for mother and baby. It is important to take the medication prescribed by your doctor regularly and follow the dosage instructions. Avoid self-medication and consult your doctor if you experience any side effects.

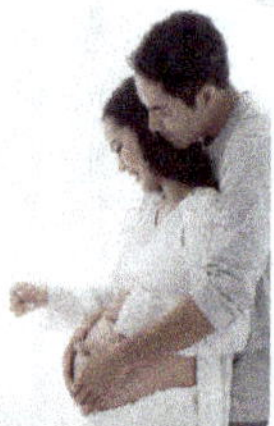

6. Fluid Consumption: Drinking enough water improves your blood circulation and helps your body to function properly. Increasing your daily water consumption can help stabilize your blood pressure. However, it is also important not to overdo your fluid intake, as too much fluid can cause edema.

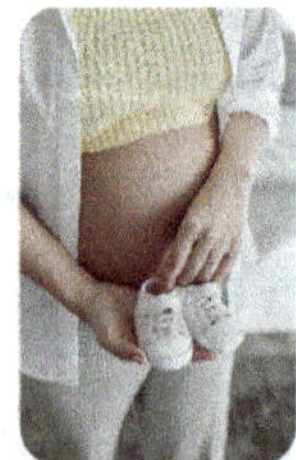
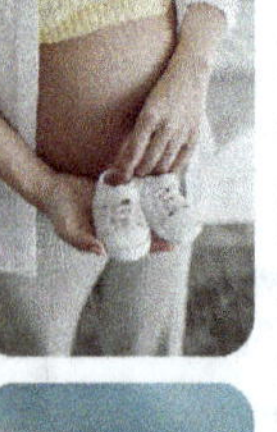

Conclusion: Controlling high blood pressure during pregnancy is critical for a healthy pregnancy and delivery. You can balance your blood pressure and prevent possible complications with a healthy diet, regular exercise, stress management and medical check-ups. By taking your doctor's recommendations into account, you can have a healthy pregnancy and ensure that your baby is born healthy.

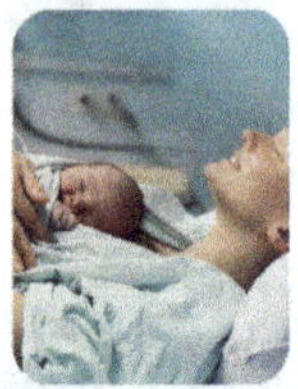

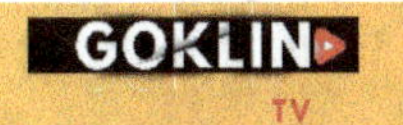

19-WHAT ARE THE RISKS OF PREMATURE BIRTH IN PREGNANCY?

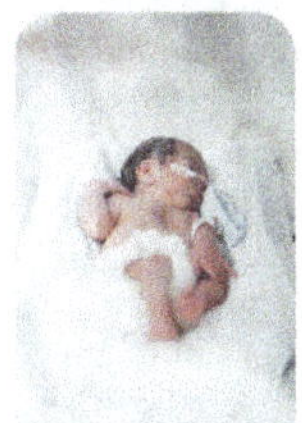

Premature birth is when a baby is born before 37 weeks of gestation. This condition carries various health risks for both the baby and the mother. Since some organs and systems of premature babies are not fully developed, they may require special care and treatment in the postnatal period. Here are some of the risks of premature birth:

1. Respiratory Problems: Since the lungs of premature babies are not fully developed, respiratory problems are common. Respiratory Distress Syndrome (RDS) is common in premature babies and may require respiratory support. Premature babies are also at increased risk of chronic lung diseases such as bronchopulmonary dysplasia (BPD).

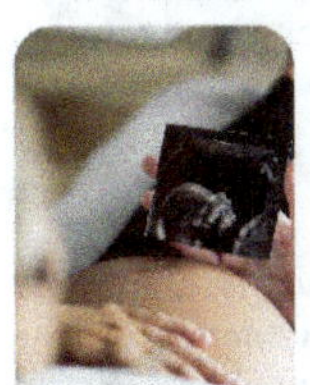

2. Brain and Nervous System Problems: Brain development accelerates in the last weeks before birth. Therefore, premature babies are at higher risk of complications such as cerebral hemorrhage (intraventricular hemorrhage) and damage to the white matter in the brain (periventricular leukomalacia). Such conditions can lead to neurological problems in the long term.

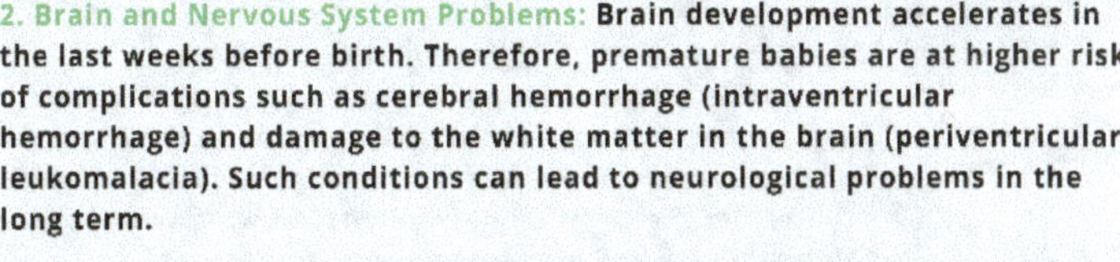

3. Digestive System Problems: Premature babies have an increased risk of a serious intestinal disease called necrotizing enterocolitis (NEC) because the intestines are not fully developed. NEC can cause damage to intestinal tissue and death. This condition requires emergency treatment and in some cases may require surgical intervention.

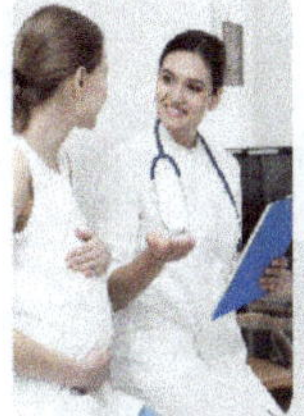

4. Immune System Weakness: Premature babies are more vulnerable to infections because their immune system is not fully developed. These babies are at risk of contracting various infections in the postnatal period, including nosocomial infections. Therefore, strict hygiene measures should be taken and babies should be protected with antibiotic treatment when necessary.

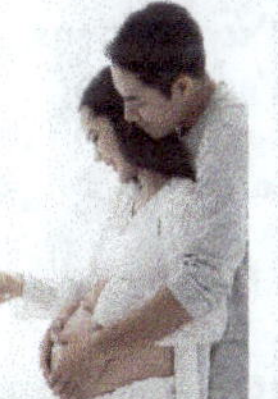

5. Vision and Hearing Problems: Babies born prematurely are at risk of an eye disease called retinopathy of prematurity (ROP) because the retina is not fully developed. If left untreated, ROP can lead to blindness. Premature babies are also at increased risk of hearing loss and should be screened for hearing after birth.

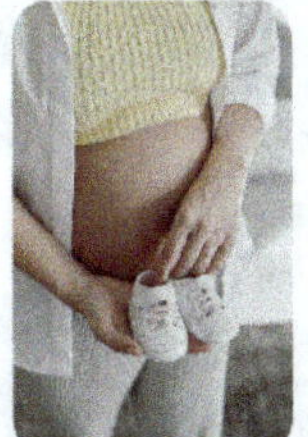

6. Long-term Developmental Problems: Premature babies may face long-term problems such as developmental delay, learning difficulties, behavioral problems and motor skill problems. Therefore, the development of children born prematurely should be closely monitored and included in early intervention programs when necessary.

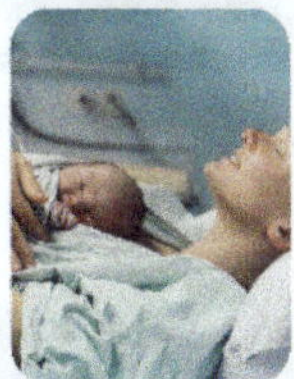

To reduce the risk of premature birth, it is important to attend regular medical check-ups during pregnancy and adopt healthy eating and lifestyle habits. Mothers at risk of preterm birth should carefully follow their doctor's recommendations and seek specialized medical care when necessary. This way, both mother and baby can have a healthy pregnancy and delivery.

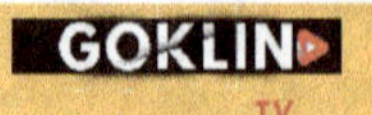

20-HOW TO PREVENT LEG SWELLİNG AND VARİCOSE VEİNS DURİNG PREGNANCY?

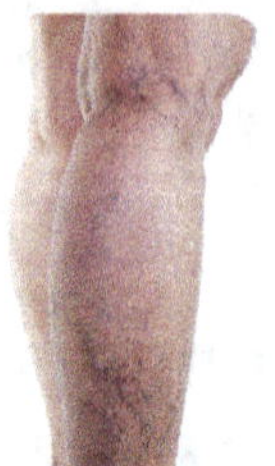

During pregnancy, the body undergoes several changes to meet the needs of the baby. One of these changes is an increase in blood volume. This can lead to swelling in the legs (edema) and varicose veins. However, there are some simple but effective ways to prevent and alleviate these conditions.

Move and Rest

Standing or sitting for long periods of time can cause blood to pool in the legs. Therefore, it is important to move at regular intervals throughout the day. Taking short walks every hour improves blood circulation and reduces swelling. Also, rest your legs by lifting them up when sitting. Supporting your legs with a pillow and lifting them above the level of the heart helps the blood return and reduces edema.

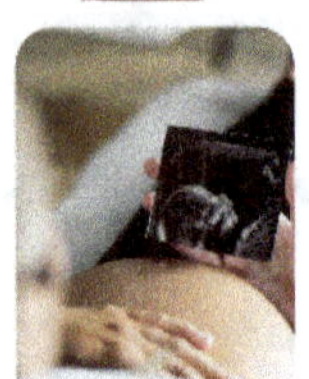

Healthy Diet and Adequate Fluid Consumption

A balanced diet can help prevent leg swelling and varicose veins. Limiting salt consumption reduces fluid retention in the body. Eating foods rich in potassium (such as bananas, spinach, avocados) helps to remove excess fluid from the body. Drinking plenty of water also maintains the body's fluid balance and prevents edema.

Use Support Socks

Compression stockings are especially useful for expectant mothers who stand or sit for long periods of time. These socks facilitate the return of blood to the heart by applying a slight pressure on the legs. These socks, which are recommended to be worn early in the day, can prevent swelling and varicose veins in the legs.

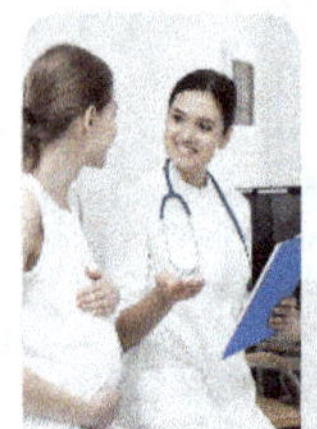
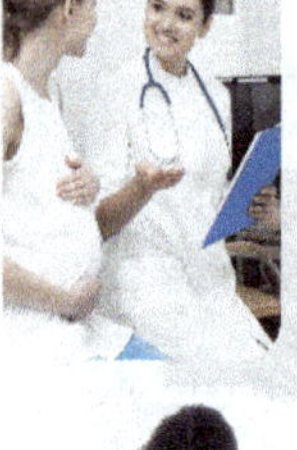

Exercise

Regular exercise improves blood circulation in the legs and strengthens the muscles. Activities such as light brisk walks, swimming and prenatal yoga maintain overall health and reduce swelling and varicose veins in the legs. At least 150 minutes of moderate-intensity exercise per week is recommended.

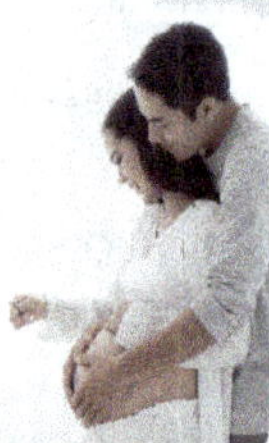

Wear Appropriate Clothing

Tight clothing can hinder blood circulation in the legs. Comfortable, loose clothing and shoes should be preferred. Also, comfortable and supportive shoes should be worn instead of high-heeled shoes.

With these recommendations, it is possible to minimize swelling and varicose veins in the legs during pregnancy. Applying these simple but effective methods to have a healthy pregnancy can make a big difference. Remember, every pregnancy is individual and you should always consult your doctor in case of any health problems.

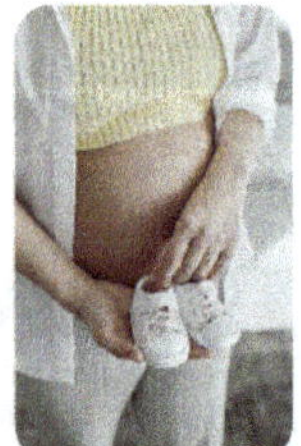
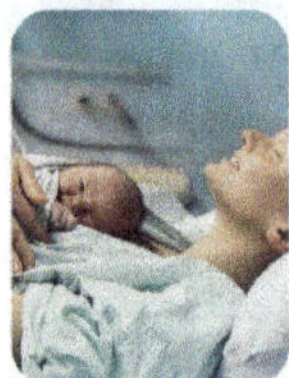

21-WHAT ARE THE COSMETICS TO AVOID DURING PREGNANCY?

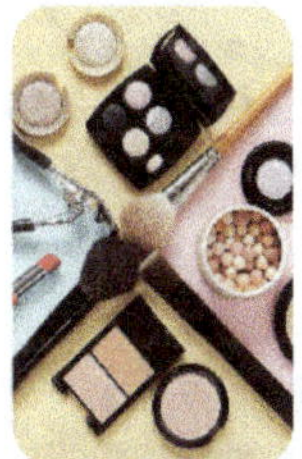

Changes in your body during pregnancy can affect not only your internal organs, but also your skin and general health. It is important to be careful with the cosmetics you use during this period, as some chemicals can harm your baby's development. Here are some cosmetics and chemicals to avoid during pregnancy:

1. Retinoids: Retinoids are ingredients commonly used in anti-aging and acne treatment. They can be found in forms such as retinol, tretinoin and isotretinoin. Retinoids can reduce wrinkles and acne by speeding up the regeneration of skin cells. However, high doses of retinoids during pregnancy may increase the risk of birth defects. Therefore, it is important to avoid products containing retinoids.

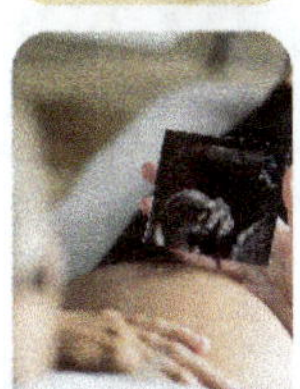

2. Salicylic Acid: Salicylic acid is another ingredient that is effective in treating acne. Although small doses are generally considered safe to use, products containing high doses of salicylic acid can be toxic when absorbed through the skin. It is best to limit or completely avoid the use of products containing salicylic acid during pregnancy.

3. Parabens: Parabens are used as preservatives in many cosmetic products. However, parabens can mimic hormones and disrupt the endocrine system. Changes in your hormone levels during pregnancy are already complicated enough, so paraben-free products should be preferred.

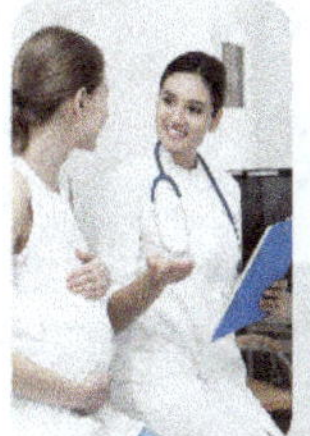

4. Phthalates: Phthalates are chemicals commonly used in cosmetics and perfumes. They preserve the fragrance and essence of products. However, phthalates can disrupt hormones and negatively affect your baby's development. Using phthalate-free products can reduce these risks.

5. Formaldehyde: Formaldehyde is found in nail hardeners and some hair care products. Formaldehyde is a known carcinogen and can be harmful if inhaled or in contact with the skin. It is important to avoid products containing formaldehyde during pregnancy.

6. Oxybenzone and Other Chemical Sunscreens: Sunscreens protect your skin from the sun's harmful UV rays. However, some chemical filters like oxybenzone can disrupt hormones. Instead, opt for physical sunscreens containing zinc oxide or titanium dioxide.

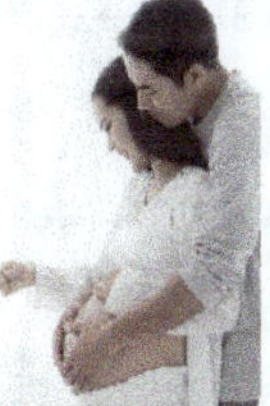

Tips for Safe Cosmetic Use

- **Read the Labels:** Read product labels carefully and choose products that do not contain the chemicals mentioned above.
- **Natural and Organic Products:** Natural and organic cosmetic products usually contain fewer harmful chemicals. However, it is important to pay attention to the ingredients of these products.
- **Consult Your Doctor:** Consult your doctor before using any cosmetic product. Your doctor can guide you on products that you can safely use during pregnancy.

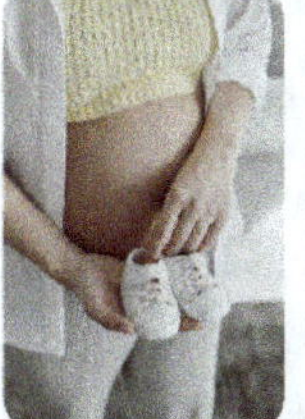

Pregnancy is a special time with many changes in your body. It is important to pay attention to the ingredients of your cosmetics to protect your health and that of your baby. By using healthy and safe products, you can protect both your beauty and your health.

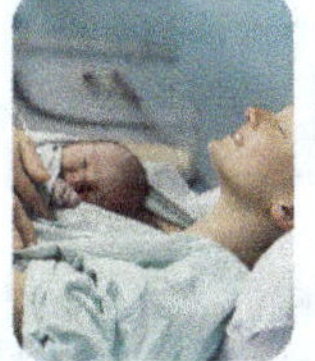

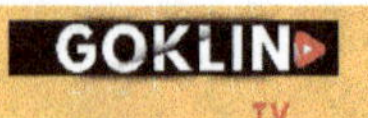

22-HAIR COLORING DURING PREGNANCY IS IT SAFE?

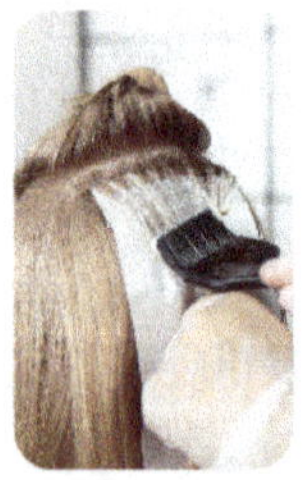

Hair coloring during pregnancy is a topic that many expectant mothers are curious about. There are concerns about whether the chemicals in hair dyes can harm the baby's development. In general, research on the safety of hair coloring during pregnancy is limited, but available data suggests that hair coloring is generally safe when certain precautions are taken.

Absorption of Chemicals

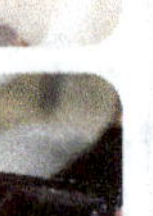

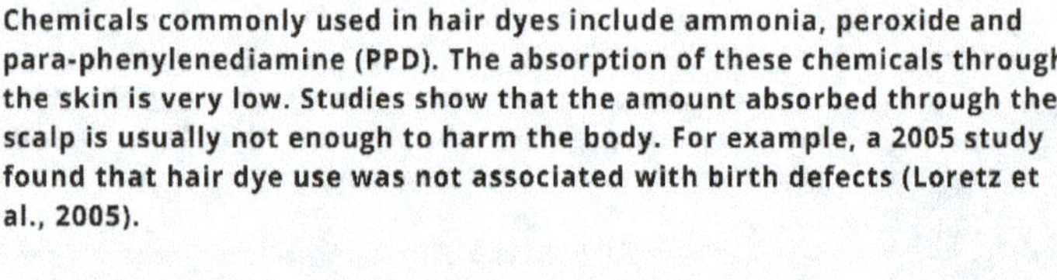

Chemicals commonly used in hair dyes include ammonia, peroxide and para-phenylenediamine (PPD). The absorption of these chemicals through the skin is very low. Studies show that the amount absorbed through the scalp is usually not enough to harm the body. For example, a 2005 study found that hair dye use was not associated with birth defects (Loretz et al., 2005).

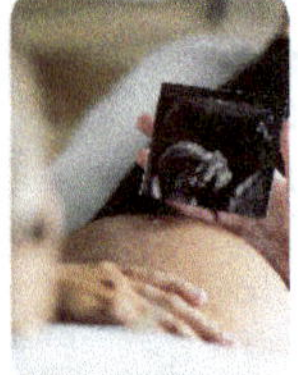

Be Careful in the First Trimester

During the first trimester of pregnancy (first trimester), the development of the baby's organs and systems is at its fastest. It is better to avoid chemical exposure during this period. The American Pregnancy Association states that it is safer to dye hair during the second and third trimesters of pregnancy.

Safe Coloring Methods

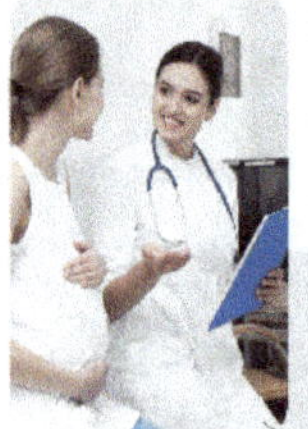

- **Herbal and Natural Dyes:** Chemical-free herbal and natural hair dyes can be preferred. Natural dyes such as henna are safer as they contain less chemicals.

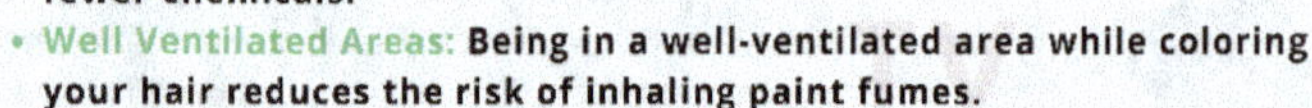

- **Semi-Permanent Dyes:** Semi-permanent or temporary dyes that do not contain ammonia and peroxide are less harmful than permanent dyes. They usually penetrate only the outer surface of the hair and contain fewer chemicals.
- **Well Ventilated Areas:** Being in a well-ventilated area while coloring your hair reduces the risk of inhaling paint fumes.
- **Glove Use:** It is important to minimize skin contact by wearing gloves when coloring.
- **Avoiding Scalp Contact:** Preventing hair dye from directly contacting the scalp reduces the absorption of chemicals. A good alternative is to apply dye to the ends of the hair or only to certain areas.

Scientific Evidence and Recommendations

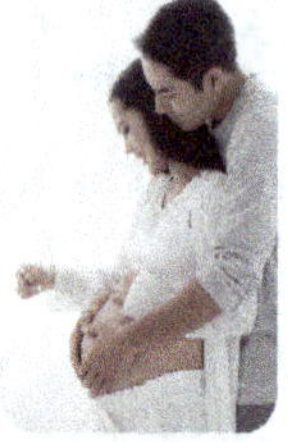

A 2013 review found that there was no definite association between hair dye and birth defects (Nohynek et al., 2013). However, in some studies, animal experiments have shown that high doses of chemicals can be harmful. Therefore, it is best to take some precautions to stay on the safe side.

Conclusion: Although hair coloring during pregnancy is generally considered safe, it is important to take some precautions and be careful. Using herbal and natural dyes, coloring in well-ventilated areas, and avoiding chemicals during the first trimester will help protect the health of both you and your baby. This way, you can protect your beauty and health at the same time. If you are considering dyeing your hair during pregnancy, it is best to talk to your doctor about it.

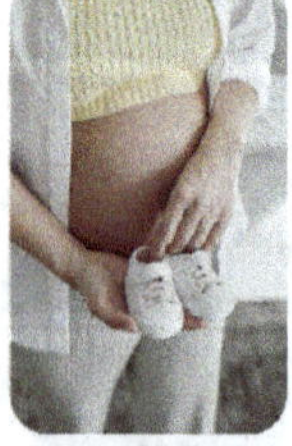

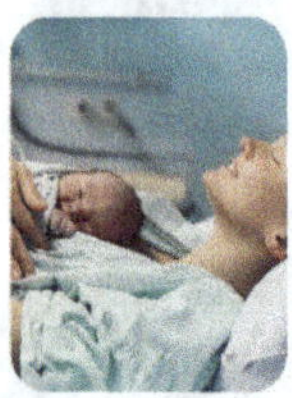

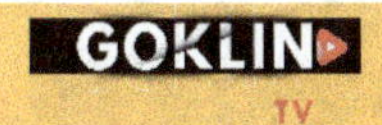

23-WHAT ARE THE SYMPTOMS OF DEPRESSION DURING PREGNANCY?

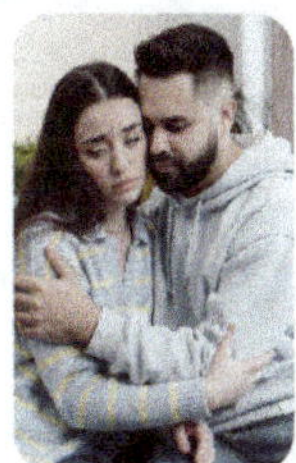

For many women, pregnancy is a time of both physical and emotional changes. It can be stressful and challenging as well as exciting. Hormonal changes, lifestyle changes and anxiety about the future during pregnancy can lead to depression in some women. Depression is a common condition during pregnancy and recognizing its symptoms is important for timely intervention.

Common Symptoms of Depression

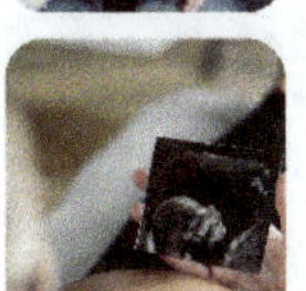

1-Feeling sad all the time: Women who experience depression during pregnancy may experience a prolonged feeling of sadness and hopelessness. This can last for most of the day and is often repeated every day.

2-Loss of Interest: No longer enjoying activities that you used to enjoy is an important symptom of depression. Hobbies, social events or daily activities may cease to interest you.

3-Fatigue and Loss of Energy: Depression can cause constant fatigue and lack of energy. Even daily tasks can become difficult and you may feel exhausted all the time.

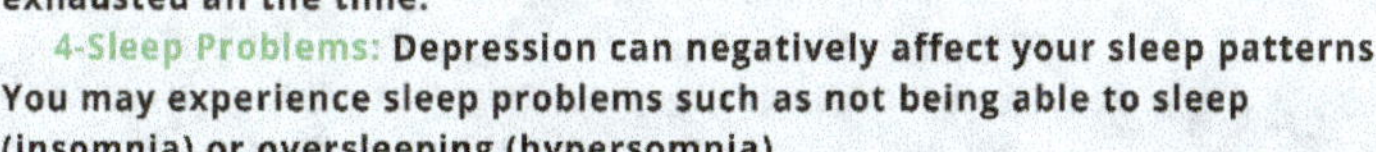
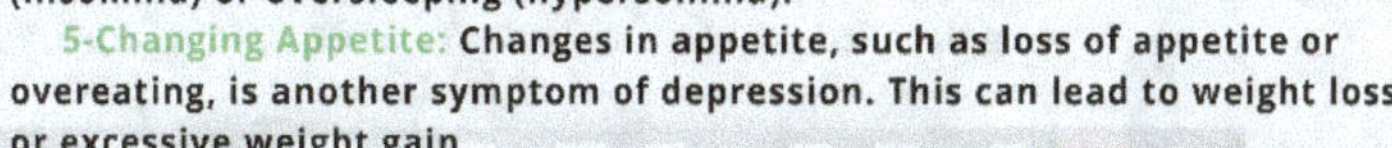

4-Sleep Problems: Depression can negatively affect your sleep patterns. You may experience sleep problems such as not being able to sleep (insomnia) or oversleeping (hypersomnia).

5-Changing Appetite: Changes in appetite, such as loss of appetite or overeating, is another symptom of depression. This can lead to weight loss or excessive weight gain.

6-Difficulty Concentrating: Concentration problems such as difficulty organizing your thoughts, forgetfulness and difficulty making decisions are common.

7-Loss of Self-Confidence: Feeling worthless, guilty or inadequate is a common symptom of depression. Such thoughts can negatively affect your overall morale and self-confidence.

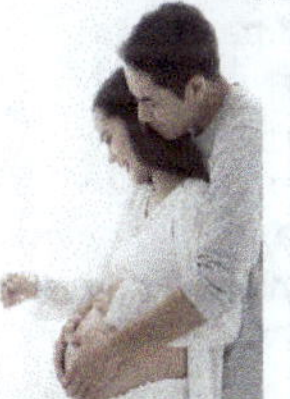

8-Physical Symptoms: Physical symptoms such as headaches, stomach problems and general pain can also be associated with depression. These symptoms often occur without a medical cause.

9-Suicidal Thoughts: In severe cases of depression, suicidal thoughts or self-harming tendencies may occur. In this case, professional help should be sought immediately.

Management and Treatment of Depression

If you are experiencing symptoms of depression during pregnancy, know that you are not alone. There are many ways to manage and treat this condition:

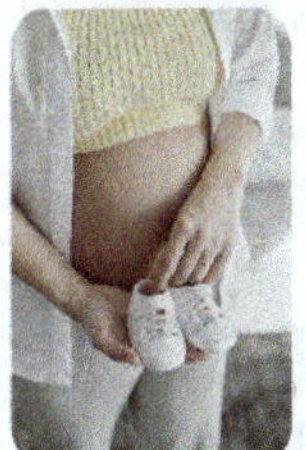

- **Support Groups and Therapy:** Psychotherapy is an effective way to manage depression. Individual therapy or support groups can help you share your feelings and learn coping strategies.
- **Medication:** In some cases, your doctor may recommend antidepressant medication. The use of medication should be done under the supervision of a doctor and after assessing the risks.
- **Healthy Lifestyle:** A balanced diet, regular exercise and adequate sleep play an important role in managing depression. In addition, relaxation techniques (such as meditation, yoga) can help reduce stress.

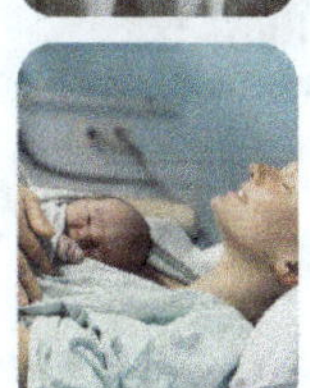

- **Social Support:** Support from family and friends can ease the emotional burden. It is important to share your feelings and seek support.

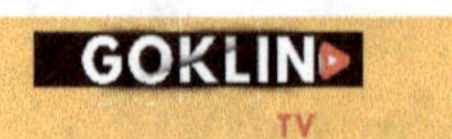

24-WHAT ARE THE COMMON INFECTIONS DURING PREGNANCY?

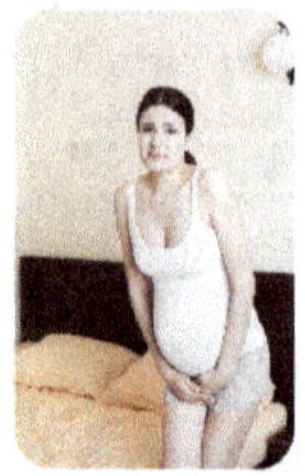

During pregnancy, susceptibility to infections can increase. The immune system undergoes changes to help the baby grow and develop, which can make some infections more easily occur. Here are some common infections during pregnancy:

1. Urinary Tract Infections (UTIs):

One of the most common infections during pregnancy, urinary tract infections can occur in the bladder, ureters or kidneys. Symptoms include frequent urination, a burning sensation when urinating, and cloudy or foul-smelling urine. Left untreated, a UTI can develop into a kidney infection and increase the risk of preterm labor. Therefore, it is important to contact your doctor when symptoms are noticed.

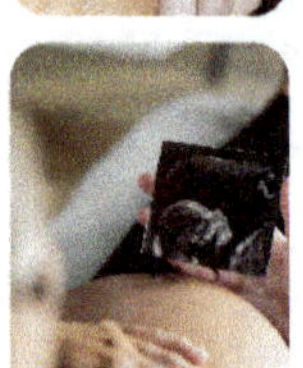

2. Bacterial Vaginosis (BV):

Bacterial vaginosis occurs when the balance of vaginal flora is disturbed. It is characterized by the growth of abnormal bacteria in the vagina. Symptoms include foul-smelling vaginal discharge, itching and burning sensation. BV can increase the risk of preterm labor and low birth weight babies. Treatment is with antibiotics.

3. Group B Streptococcus (GBS):

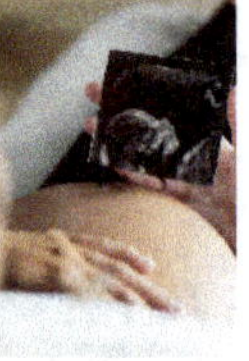

GBS is a bacteria found in the intestine and genital area. It is usually asymptomatic during pregnancy, but can be passed to the baby during labor and cause serious infections. A screening test at 35-37 weeks of pregnancy can detect the presence of GBS. If it is positive, antibiotic treatment is administered during labor.

4. Toxoplasmosis:

Toxoplasmosis is caused by infection with the parasite Toxoplasma gondii. It can be transmitted through consumption of raw or undercooked meat and contact with infected cat feces. If infected during pregnancy, it can cause serious birth defects or infections in the baby. To avoid this infection, it is important to consume well-cooked meat and be careful when cleaning cat litter.

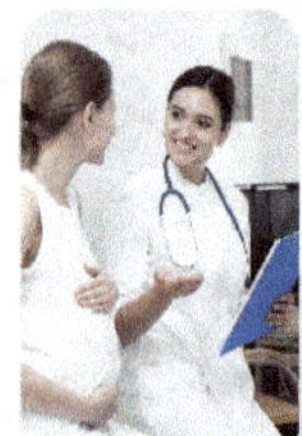

5. Cytomegalovirus (CMV):

CMV is a common virus belonging to the herpes virus family. It usually causes no symptoms, but if infected during pregnancy, it can be passed to the baby and cause birth defects or developmental problems. Good hygiene practices (for example, washing hands frequently) are important to prevent infection.

6. Influenza:

The flu virus can cause serious illness in pregnant women. Getting a flu vaccine during pregnancy helps protect both mother and baby. Flu symptoms include high fever, cough, sore throat, body aches and tiredness. Flu is treated with antiviral medicines and supportive care.

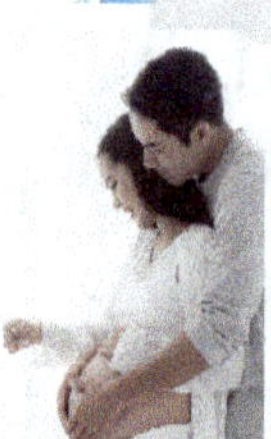

Prevention and Treatment:

The best way to prevent infections during pregnancy is to practice good hygiene. Hands should be washed frequently, consumption of raw or undercooked meat should be avoided and doctor-recommended vaccination schedules should be followed. Contacting a health professional immediately when signs of infection are recognized is critical to protect the health of both mother and baby.

By paying attention to these measures to minimize the risk of infection during pregnancy, you can have a healthy pregnancy.

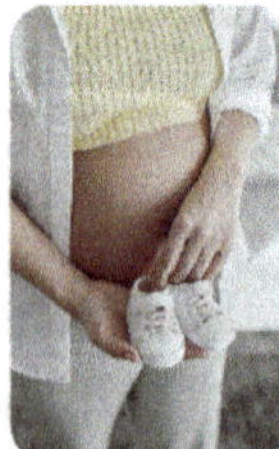

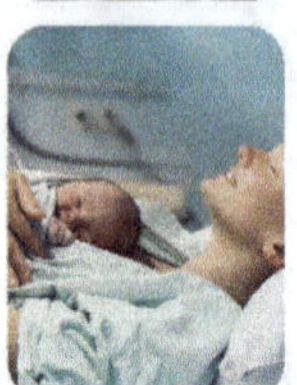

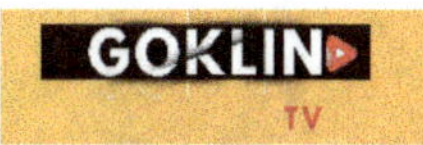

25-WHAT METHODS OF DELİVERY ARE AVAİLABLE?

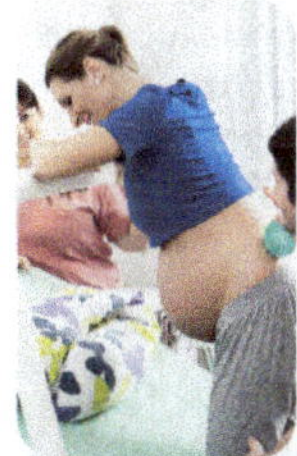

Childbirth is the process of bringing a baby into the world and there are a variety of birth methods to accomplish this process. Each method of delivery is chosen depending on factors such as the health of the mother and baby, the progress of the birth process and personal preferences. Here are the most common methods of childbirth:

1. Vaginal delivery:

Vaginal birth is the most common method of delivery. The mother gives birth by pushing the baby through the vaginal canal. This method of delivery is usually the safest for mother and baby. The advantages of vaginal birth include a faster recovery time, a shorter hospital stay and a lower risk of breathing problems for the baby. However, in some cases, the birth process can be long and difficult.

2. Caesarean section (C-section):

A caesarean section is the surgical removal of the baby from the womb. A caesarean section can be planned or performed in emergency situations. Planned cesarean section may be preferred for reasons such as the mother's health status, the position of the baby or twin pregnancy. An emergency caesarean section is performed when complications arise during labor. Cesarean section has a longer recovery time than vaginal delivery and carries surgical risks.

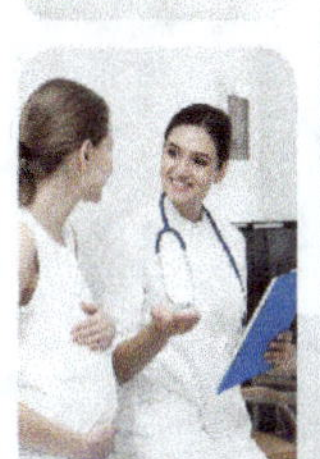

3. Epidural Delivery:

Epidural delivery involves the use of epidural anesthesia for pain management during vaginal delivery. An epidural is a local anesthetic given through a catheter placed in the lumbar region. This method significantly reduces the mother's pain during labor. The epidural keeps the mother conscious and helps her to have a more comfortable birth. However, in some cases, epidural side effects or complications may occur.

4. Water birth:

Water birth involves the mother giving birth in water in a birthing pool or bathtub. This method can reduce labor pains and facilitate the birth process thanks to the relaxing effect of water. Water birth can take place both at home and in a hospital. However, the doctor should decide whether this method is suitable for all expectant mothers.

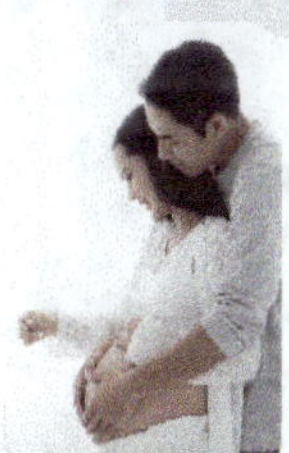

5. Natural childbirth:

Natural childbirth is birth without medical interventions or pain medication. This method encourages the mother to trust her body and the birth process. In natural childbirth, the mother has freedom of movement and the possibility to use different birthing positions. Natural birth usually takes place in birth centers or at home and is supported by a trained midwife or doula.

6. Assisted Birth with Vacuum or Forceps:

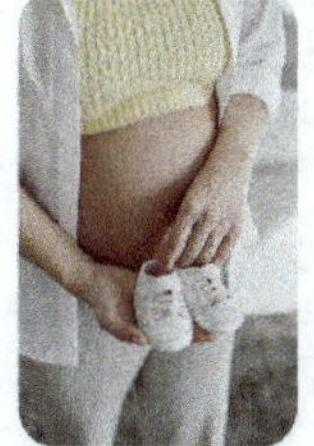

Vacuum or forceps-assisted birth are methods used when the baby is stuck in the birth canal. The vacuum pulls the baby through a device placed on the baby's head, while forceps are used to help pull the baby out of the birth canal using metal instruments. These methods may be necessary for the baby's health in the final stages of labor.

Conclusion:

Each method of delivery is chosen depending on factors such as the health of the mother and baby, the course of labor and the mother's preferences. When planning your birth, it is important to discuss all the options with your doctor and choose the method that suits you best. Being informed about how the birth process will go will help you spend this special moment in a safer and more comfortable way.

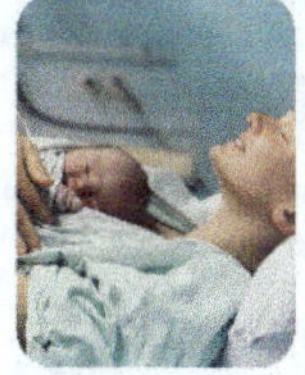

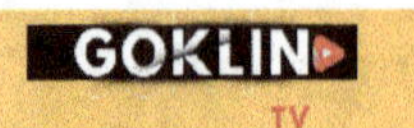

26-HOW MUCH SHOULD WEİGHT GAİN BE DURİNG PREGNANCY?

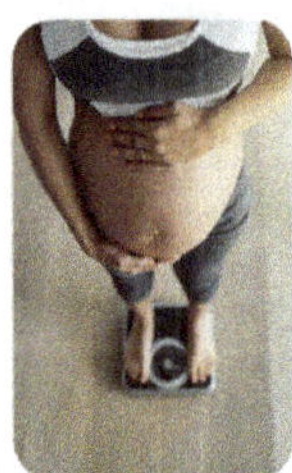

Weight gain during pregnancy is of great importance for the health of both mother and baby. This weight gain should be balanced and healthy. How much weight should be gained depends on the pre-pregnancy body mass index (BMI) and general health.

WHAT İS BODY MASS İNDEX (BMI)?

Body mass index (BMI) is a measure of a person's weight in relation to their height. BMI is calculated as body weight in kilograms divided by the square of height in meters. For example, the BMI of a woman who weighs 70 kilograms and is 1.65 meters tall is calculated as follows:

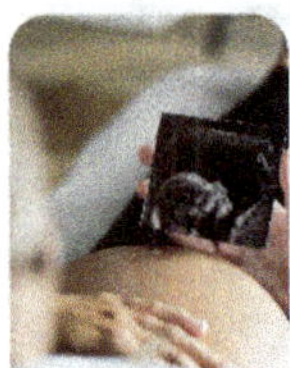

$$BMI = \frac{70}{1.65^2} = 25.7$$

In this case, the woman's BMI is 25.7, which falls into the overweight category.

BMI and Weight Gain Before Pregnancy:

1-Normal Weight (BMI 18.5 - 24.9):
- Ideal weight gain: 11-16 kg
- Women of normal weight should gain weight within this range for a healthy pregnancy. This amount is needed for the baby to grow and to meet the mother's energy needs.

2-Low Weight (BMI < 18.5):
- Ideal weight gain: 12-18 kg
- Women who are underweight should gain more weight during pregnancy. This is necessary to support the baby's development.

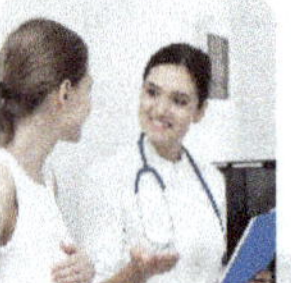

3-Overweight (BMI 25 - 29.9):
- Ideal weight gain: 7-11 kg
- Women who are overweight should limit their weight gain. This is important to reduce the risk of pregnancy-related complications.

4-Obesity (BMI ≥ 30):
- Ideal weight gain: 5-9 kg
- Obese women should gain less weight during pregnancy. This reduces the risk of complications such as gestational diabetes and pre-eclampsia.

Weight Gain by Trimester:

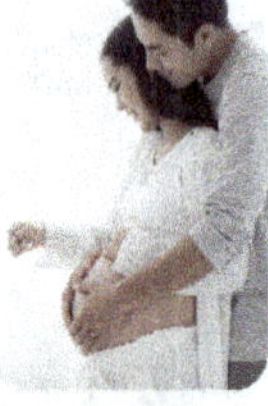

1st Trimester (First 12 Weeks):
- Weight gain during the first trimester is usually around 1-2 kg. Some women may not gain or lose weight during this period due to morning sickness and loss of appetite. This is normal and usually not a concern.

2nd Trimester (13-27 weeks):
- Weight gain accelerates during this period. On average, it is expected to gain about 0.5 kg per week. This is a period when the baby is growing rapidly and the mother's body is preparing for childbirth and breastfeeding.

3rd Trimester (28-40 weeks):
- Weight gain continues at the same pace as in the second trimester. The baby grows and gains more weight during this period. A gain of about 0.5 kg per week is normal.

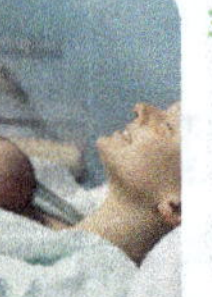

26-HOW MUCH SHOULD WEİGHT GAİN BE DURİNG PREGNANCY?

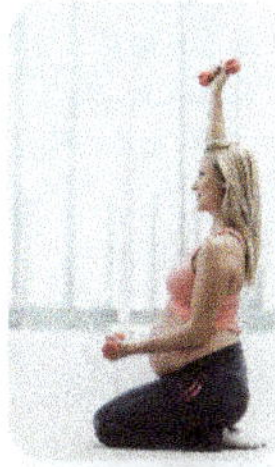

Factors Affecting Weight Gain:
- **Nutrition:** A balanced and nutritious diet supports healthy weight gain. It is important to eat plenty of fruits, vegetables, whole grains, protein and healthy fats.
- **Exercise:** Regular and light exercise (walking, swimming, etc.) can help control weight and make pregnancy more comfortable.
- **Fluid Consumption:** Drinking enough water maintains the body's water balance and controls weight gain.

Example:

Ayşe is a woman who weighed 60 kilograms and was 1.65 meters tall before pregnancy. Her BMI is calculated as follows:

$$BMI = \frac{60}{1.65^2} = 22$$

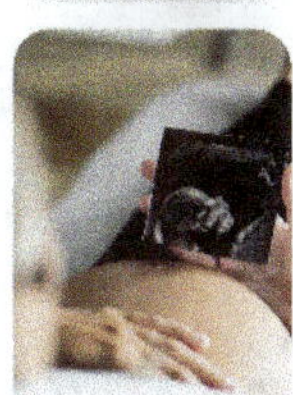

In this case, Ayşe falls into the normal weight category. For a healthy weight gain during her pregnancy, she is expected to gain between 11-16 kilograms. Starting with a weight gain of 1-2 kilograms in the first trimester, she should gain about 0.5 kilograms per week in the second and third trimesters.

Conclusion:

Healthy weight gain during pregnancy is critical for the health of both mother and baby. It is important to remember that weight gain can vary depending on pre-pregnancy body mass index and general health. Regularly checking your weight gain with your doctor and adopting healthy eating and exercise habits will help you have a healthy pregnancy.

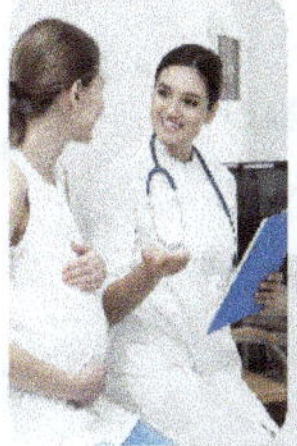

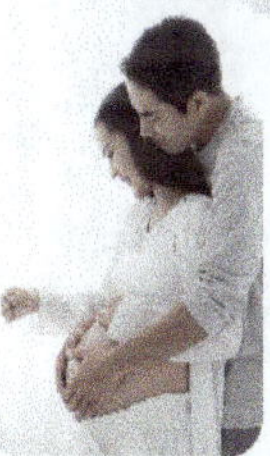

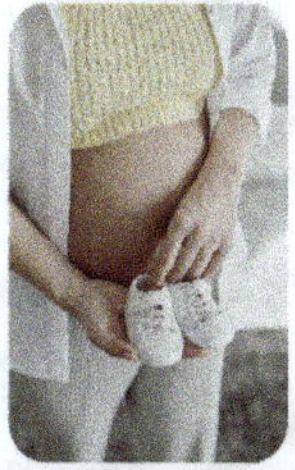

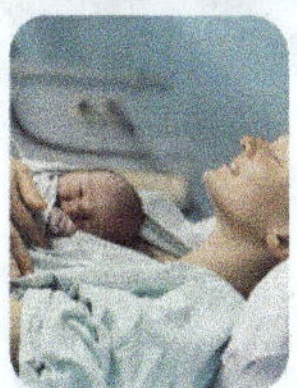

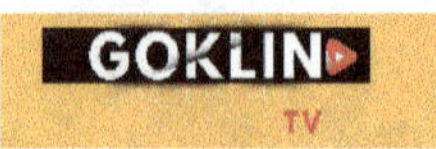

27-HOW TO PREPARE THE BABY'S ROOM DURİNG PREGNANCY?

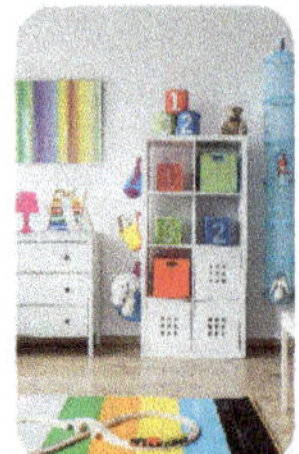

Preparing the baby's room is an exciting process for parents. In this process, the safety and comfort of the baby should be prioritized. Let's look at a few important points on how to prepare the baby's room with scientific approaches.

Safety is Priority

The most important issue when preparing a baby's room is safety. Furniture should be sturdy and secured against tipping. When choosing a crib, check whether it complies with international safety standards. The space between the crib railings should not be wider than 6 cm so that the baby does not get stuck. Also, avoid soft mattresses and pillows, as these can increase the risk of suffocation.

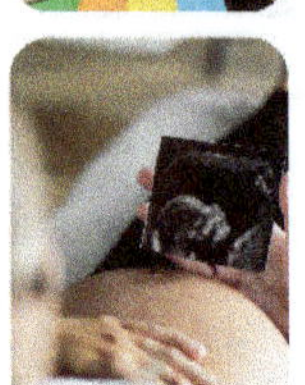

Air Quality and Temperature

Air quality is important in the baby's room. The room should be ventilated regularly. Chemical-free paints with low VOC (volatile organic compounds) should be preferred. The room temperature should be kept between 20-22°C and humidity should be 40-60%. These conditions allow the baby to breathe easily and prevent dry skin.

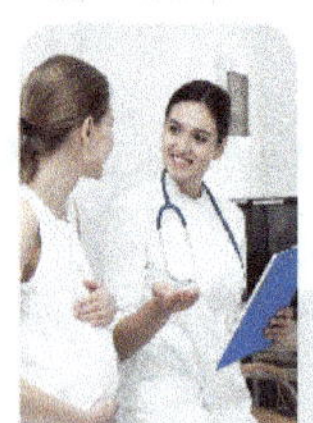
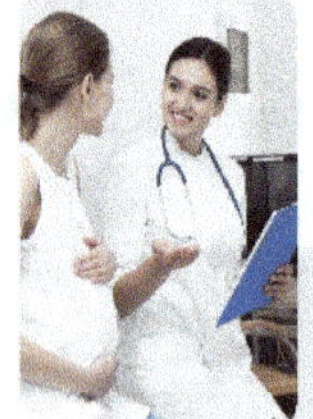

Lighting

Natural light is ideal for a baby's room. However, arrangements should be made so that sunlight does not directly hit the bed. Using a dim night light for the night can help the baby's sleep patterns and provide convenience for parents during night feedings.

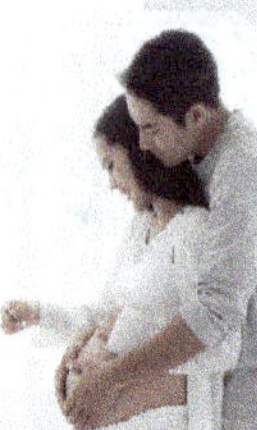

Ergonomic and Functional Design

Ergonomic arrangements should be made in the baby room to meet the needs of the parents. There should be easy access between the crib, changing table and cupboards. Baby care products should be easily accessible on the changing table. These arrangements both facilitate the parents' work and increase the safety of the baby.

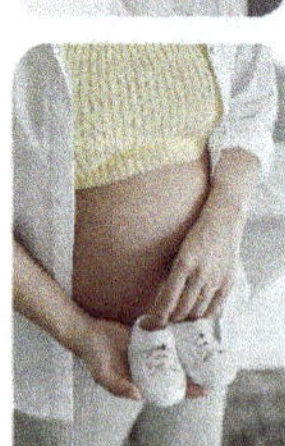

Cleaning and Hygiene

The cleanliness and hygiene of the baby's room is also very important. The room should be cleaned regularly and free of dust. The use of carpets or rugs should be limited because they can accumulate dust and allergens. Baby clothes and bedding should be washed with hypoallergenic detergents.

With these recommendations, you can make the baby's room both safe and comfortable. With scientific approaches and practical arrangements, you can create an ideal environment to support your baby's development. Above all, creating a loving environment that suits your baby's needs will contribute to their healthy and happy growth.

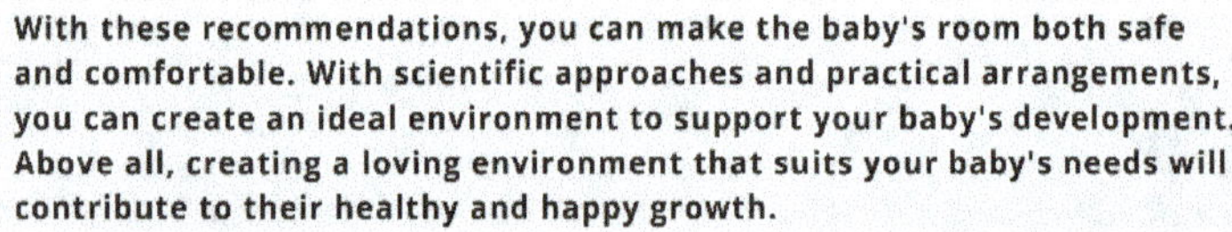
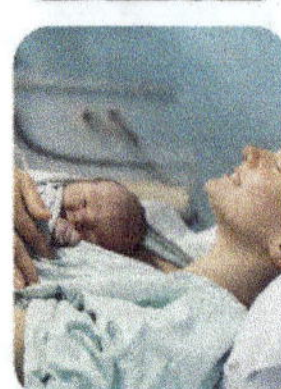
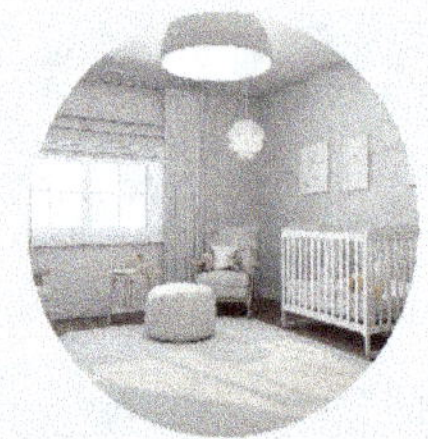
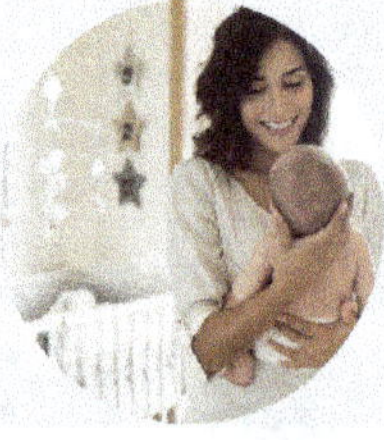
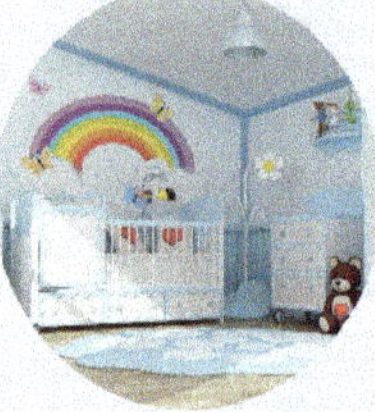

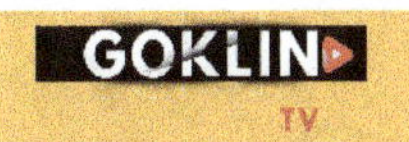

27-HOW TO PREPARE THE BABY'S ROOM DURING PREGNANCY?

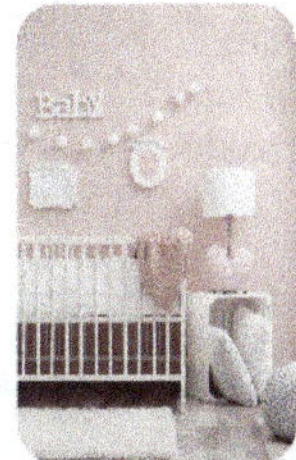

BABY ROOM DESIGN
Safety Prioritized Furniture

- **The cradle:** Place it in a central place in the room. The crib should be at least 30 cm away from walls and other furniture. The space between the crib railings should not be wider than 6 cm.
- **Changing Table:** Place it close to the crib. So you don't have to move much when changing the baby. Place baby care products in an organized manner on the changing table.
- **Cabinets and Drawers:** Secure furniture to the wall to prevent it from tipping over. Place cabinets and drawers close to the crib and changing table for easy access.

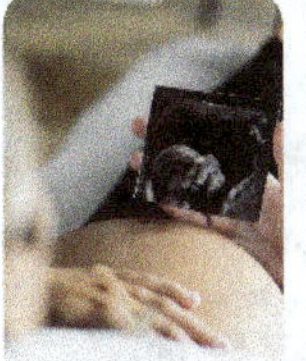

Air Quality and Heat

- **Ventilation:** Open the windows and doors of the room regularly to let in fresh air. Remember to install security locks around the windows.
- **Paints:** Color the room using low-VOC, chemical-free paints. The overall color of the room can be light and pastel tones.
- **Heater and Humidifier:** Use a safe heater to keep the room temperature between 20-22°C. Install a humidifier to keep the humidity between 40-60%.

Lighting.

- **Natural Light:** Make sure the room gets plenty of natural light. Keep the curtains open to let in sunlight, but be careful not to direct sunlight into the crib.
- **Night Light:** Use a dim night light for nighttime feedings and care. Place the lamp close to the crib.

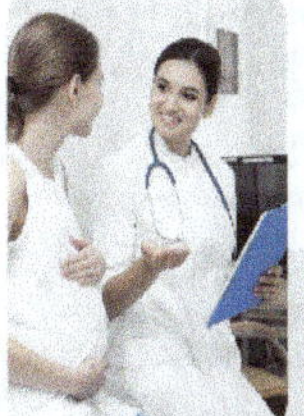

Ergonomic and Functional Design

- **Layout Layout:** Arrange the crib, changing table and cupboards for easy access. This layout makes baby care easier and saves time for parents.
- **Shelves and Baskets:** Create an organized environment by using wall-mounted shelves and baskets for baby care products, toys and clothes.

Cleaning and Hygiene

- **Flooring:** Limit the use of carpets or rugs on the room floor. Instead, choose an easy-to-clean floor material.
- **Cleaning Products:** Wash baby clothes and bedding with hypoallergenic detergents. Dust and clean the room regularly.

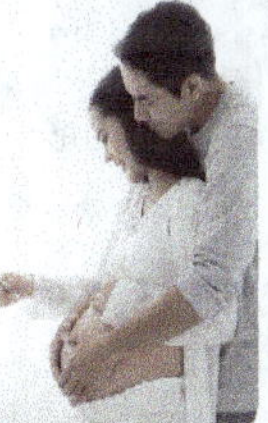
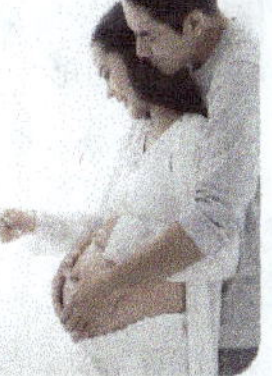

Visualization

- **Colors and Decoration:** Light pastel tones can be used on walls and furniture. For example, colors such as light blue, pastel pink, mint green provide a calming and fresh environment.
- **Accessories:** Simple and safe decorations such as cute animal figures or star patterns on the wall can be used. Soft and hypoallergenic materials should be preferred for textiles such as curtains, baby blankets and cushions.

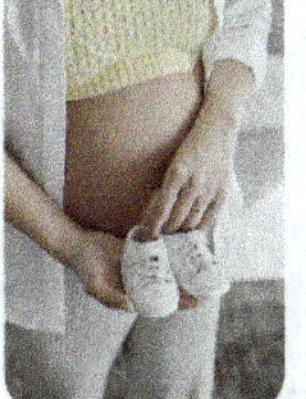

With this design guide, you can prepare the baby's room in a safe and healthy way based on scientific principles and create an aesthetically pleasing environment.

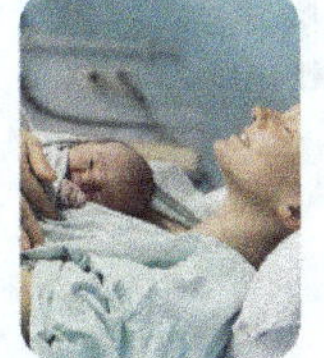

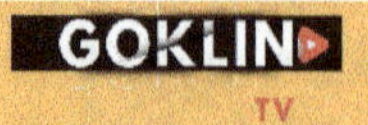

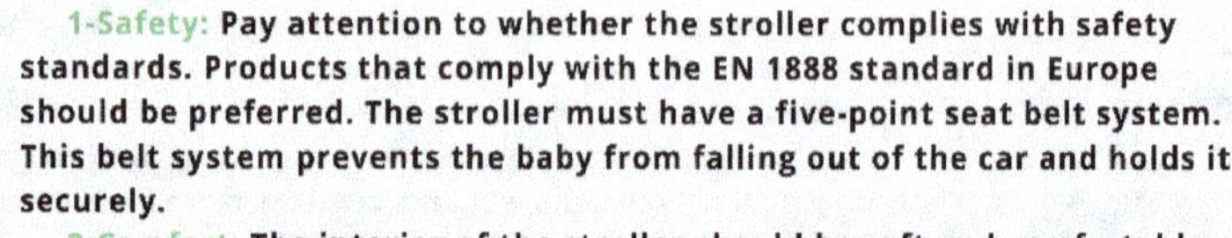

28-HOW TO CHOOSE A STROLLER AND OTHER BABY PRODUCTS?

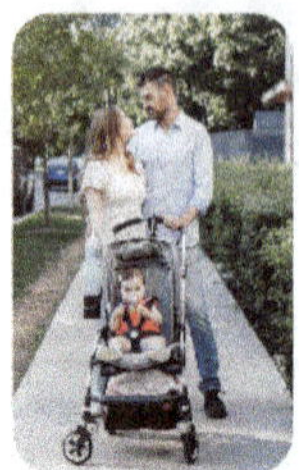

When choosing strollers and other baby products, it is important to consider the needs of both the baby and the parents. Here are some scientific and practical tips to consider when choosing these products:

Choosing a Baby Stroller

1-Safety: Pay attention to whether the stroller complies with safety standards. Products that comply with the EN 1888 standard in Europe should be preferred. The stroller must have a five-point seat belt system. This belt system prevents the baby from falling out of the car and holds it securely.

2-Comfort: The interior of the stroller should be soft and comfortable. The adjustable back support ensures that your baby is comfortable while sleeping. Pillows and cushions that support the baby's head and neck are also an important detail.

3-Ease of Use: The fact that the stroller is foldable and lightweight provides a great advantage, especially in urban use. The fact that the stroller can be easily transported and can fit in the car makes parents' daily life easier.

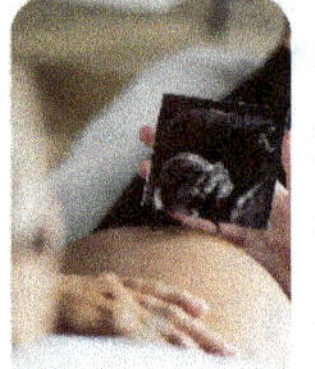

4-Wheels and Suspension: The wheels of the stroller should be large and durable. The suspension system prevents the baby from shaking on bumpy roads and provides a comfortable journey.

Other Baby Products Selection

1-Baby Diaper: Cotton and hypoallergenic diapers should be preferred. These diapers do not irritate the baby's sensitive skin and offer a comfortable use. When choosing between disposable and washable diapers, you should consider the advantages and disadvantages of both types.

2-Bottle and Pacifier: BPA-free plastic or glass baby bottles should be preferred. These products are safer for the baby's health. It is also important that the pacifiers are made of silicone or rubber materials and have an orthodontic design.

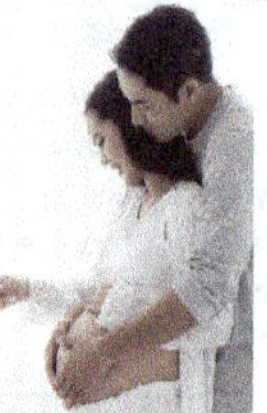

3-Baby Carrying Bag: An ergonomically designed baby carrier bag protects parents' spine health. Adjustable straps and supportive belts distribute the baby's weight evenly and provide comfortable transportation.

4-Baby Clothes: Cotton, breathable and hypoallergenic clothes should be preferred. Clothes that do not irritate the baby's skin and are easy to put on and take off are ideal for daily use. It is also important that the clothes are washable and durable.

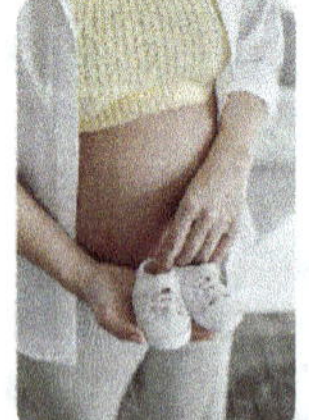

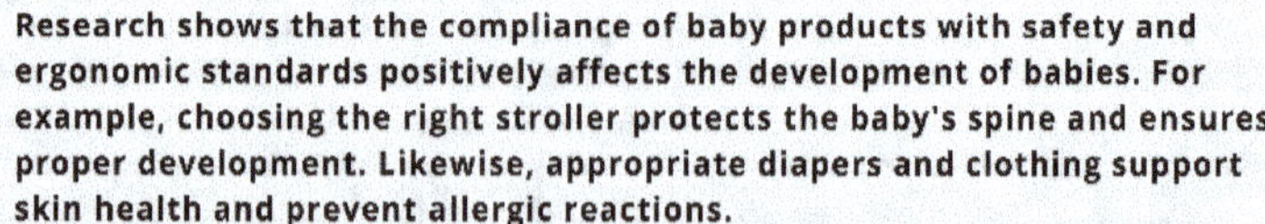

Scientific Perspective

Research shows that the compliance of baby products with safety and ergonomic standards positively affects the development of babies. For example, choosing the right stroller protects the baby's spine and ensures proper development. Likewise, appropriate diapers and clothing support skin health and prevent allergic reactions.

By prioritizing quality and safety when choosing baby products, you can ensure the comfort of both your baby and you. With these scientific and practical tips, you can shop for baby products with confidence.

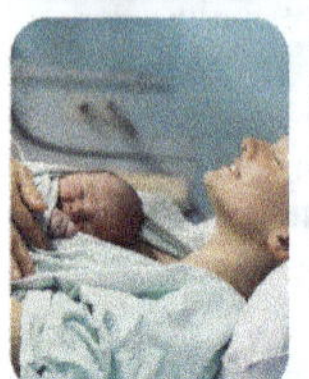

29-WHEN DO BİRTH PAİNS START?

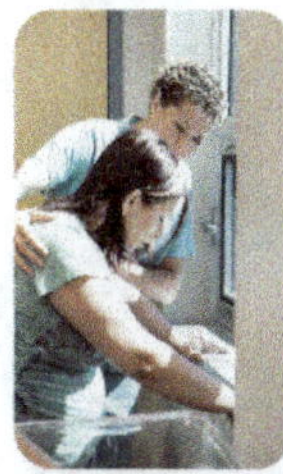

Labour pains are characterized by regular contractions of the uterus, which signal the start of labour. They usually start in late pregnancy, as the baby moves into the birth canal. The timing of the onset of labor pains can vary with each pregnancy, but they usually start close to the due date.

When labor contractions start:
Between Weeks 37-42:
Labor contractions usually start between 37 and 42 weeks of pregnancy. This period is called "term" and the baby is fully ready for birth. Most babies are born during this time.
Birth Symptoms:
-The onset of labor can be marked by various symptoms. These include regular and increasingly strong contractions, the breaking of water (discharge of amniotic fluid) and increased vaginal discharge.
-Contractions may be irregular at first, but become more regular and frequent as labor approaches.

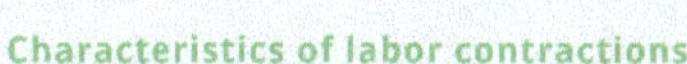

Characteristics of labor contractions:
Braxton Hicks contractions:
Braxton Hicks contractions are contractions that start weeks or even months before labor, known as "false labor contractions". Unlike real contractions, these contractions are irregular and usually go away with rest or a change of position.
Real labor contractions:
Real contractions are regular and rhythmic. Each contraction lasts about 30-70 seconds and becomes more frequent and more intense over time. These contractions usually start in the lower back and spread to the abdomen.

Management of Labor Pains:
Mild Contractions:
In the early stages of labor, contractions are usually mild and tolerable. During this period, taking a walk, taking a warm shower or practicing relaxation techniques can ease contractions.

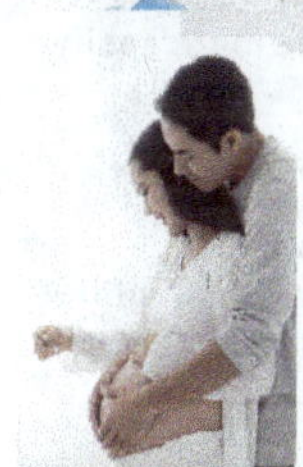

More Severe Contractions:
When contractions become more severe, it is time to go to the hospital or birth center for delivery. It is important to communicate with your doctor or midwife at this stage.
Pain Management:
There are various options for pain management during labour, such as epidural anesthesia, a birth pool, breathing techniques or drug-free methods. You can discuss with your doctor which method is best for you.

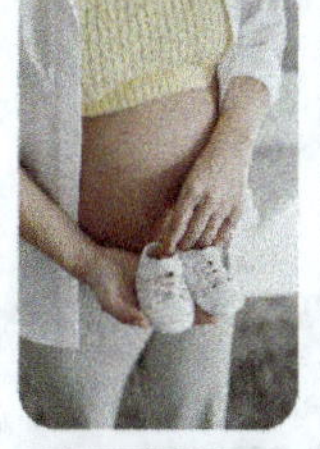

Conclusion
The timing of the onset of contractions varies for each woman, but they usually start late in pregnancy, between 37 and 42 weeks. Symptoms such as regular and intensifying contractions, water breaking and increased vaginal discharge are signs that labor has started. When labor begins, it is important to communicate with your doctor or midwife to manage the contractions and ensure a safe delivery. Relaxation techniques and pain management methods can help to alleviate labor pains.

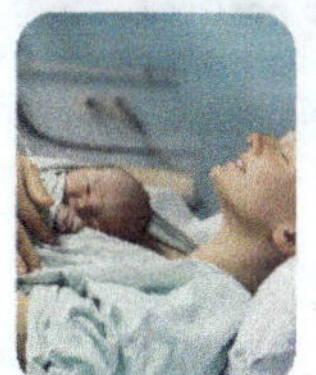

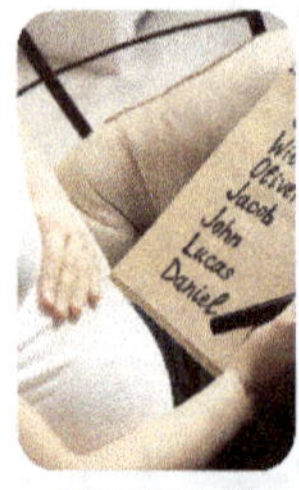

Choosing a baby name is an exciting and important process for new parents. The name will play an important role in the child's identity and life. Various scientific and cultural factors should be taken into consideration when choosing a name. Here are some important points to consider when choosing a baby name:

1. Cultural and Familial Context:

A name should be compatible with cultural and familial roots. Names that have an important place in the family and culture can have a strong place in the child's identity. For example, names that are frequently used in the family or names that are culturally meaningful may be preferred.

2. Meaning and Origin:

The meaning and origin of the name are important factors affecting the choice. Scientific research shows that names have psychological effects on people. Names with positive meanings can increase a child's self-confidence and social acceptance.

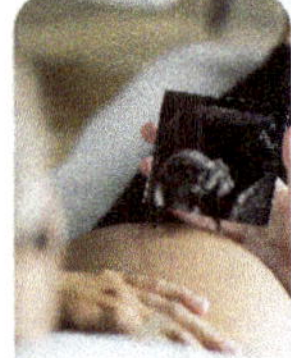

3. Ease of Pronunciation and Spelling:

The name should be easy to pronounce and spell. Names with difficult pronunciation or complicated spelling can cause difficulties in the child's life. According to scientific studies, names that are easy to pronounce can have positive effects on social acceptance and academic achievement.

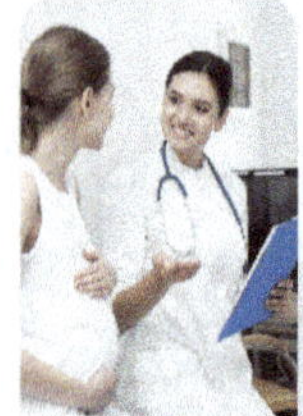
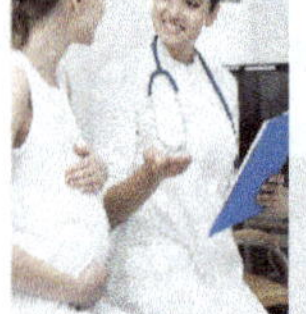

4. Social and Psychological Effects of Names:

Research on the social and psychological effects of names shows how names are perceived and evaluated in individuals' lives. For example, names that are widely known and liked may help a child to be more easily accepted in their social environment.

5. Unic and Traditional Names:

Unic (unique) names can give a child a sense of difference and individuality, while traditional names can strengthen cultural and familial ties. Scientific studies suggest that unique names can provide social and professional advantages in some cases.

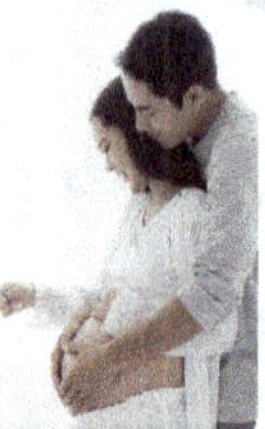

6. Emotional and Aesthetic Factors:

Parents' emotional ties and aesthetic preferences also play an important role in name choice. The name can carry an emotional meaning for the parents, which can give the child a special place in their life.

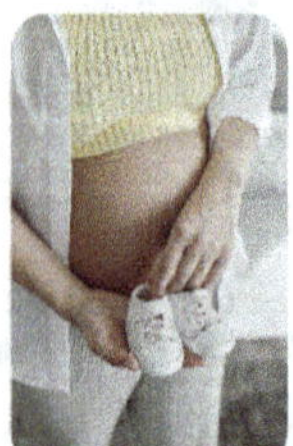
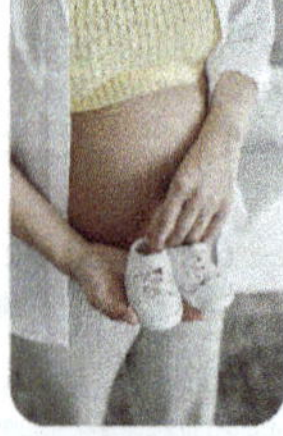

Conclusion:

Choosing a baby name should take into account cultural, familial, psychological and aesthetic factors. Scientifically based criteria such as the meaning, pronunciation, spelling and social impact of names help to make a healthy and informed choice. Names that will have a positive impact on the child's identity should be chosen, taking into account the emotional attachment and aesthetic preferences of the parents.

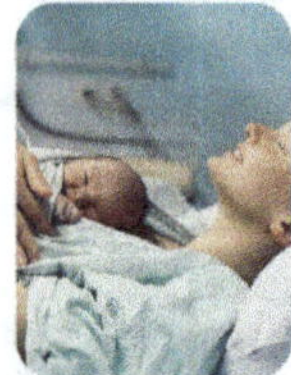

POSTPARTUM (10 QUESTİONS)
Let's Explore Together!

1-HOW LONG DOES POSTPARTUM RECOVERY TAKE?

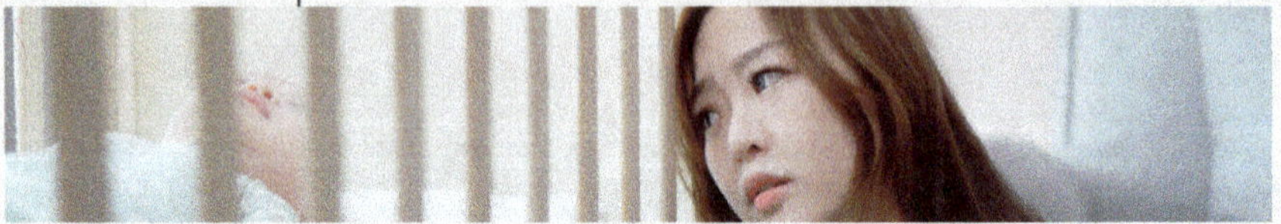

The recovery period after childbirth varies for each woman, but in general there are certain stages. Knowing these stages can make it easier to understand the process.

First week
Immediately after the birth, your body starts to recover.

- **Bleeding and discharge:** During the first few weeks, you may have vaginal bleeding (lochia) and discharge. This indicates that your uterus is healing.
- **Cramps:** You may feel mild cramps as your uterus tries to return to its original size. This process can take up to 6 weeks.

First 6 weeks
This is the time when your body is largely recovering.

- **Stitches:** If you had an episiotomy during normal labor or a caesarean section, the stitches usually heal within 2-3 weeks. However, full healing can take several months.
- **Energy Level:** It is normal to feel tired in the first weeks. Paying attention to rest and sleep will speed up your recovery.

First 3 months
In the first 3 months, your body and hormones begin to stabilize.

- **Hormonal Changes:** You may experience emotional fluctuations as your hormonal balance tries to return to normal. Postpartum depression is common and it is important to seek support.
- **Breastfeeding:** Breastfeeding requires a period of adjustment for both you and your baby. During this period, there may be problems such as nipple sores or blocked milk ducts.

6 Months and After
After six months, most women feel physically better.

- **Energy Level:** Your energy level increases as your sleep pattern settles.
- **Weight Loss:** It may take time to lose the weight gained during pregnancy. You can speed up this process with gentle exercise and a healthy diet.

Full recovery can take up to a year. Every woman's recovery is different, so it is important to take good care of yourself and follow your doctor's advice. Be patient and give your body time.

2-WHAT ARE BREASTFEEDİNG TECHNİQUES AND POSİTİONS?

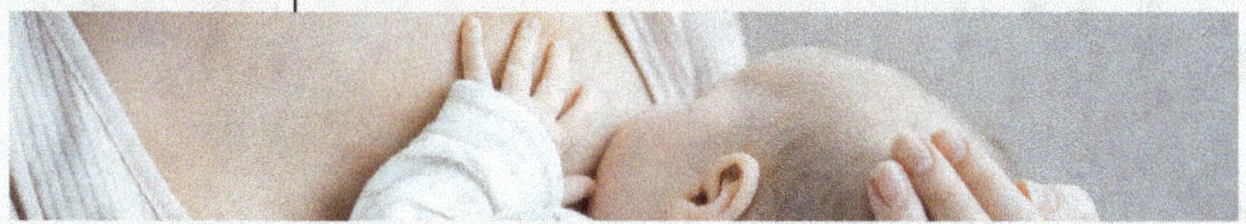

Breastfeeding helps to create a special bond between mother and baby and is important for the healthy growth of the baby. The right breastfeeding techniques and positions ensure that both mother and baby are comfortable and make the breastfeeding process more efficient.

Breastfeeding Techniques

1-Positioning the baby correctly: It is important that your baby opens its mouth wide and fully grasps the nipple. Your baby's lower lip should be facing outwards and should have a good grip on the breast tissue inside the mouth. This ensures that your baby gets enough milk and prevents the formation of nipple cracks.

2-Frequent and Regular Breastfeeding: In the first few weeks, your baby should be breastfed every 2-3 hours. This helps your milk production to increase and your baby's weight gain to be regular. Breastfeeding both breasts for equal amounts of time balances milk production.

BREASTFEEDİNG POSİTİONS

1 - Cradle Position:

In this classic position, you place your baby in the crook of your arm and rest his or her head in the crook of your elbow. You can support your breast with your other hand. This position is especially suitable for newborn babies.

2-Cross Cradle Position:

It is the opposite of the cradle position. You switch arms while holding your baby, i.e. you use your left arm when breastfeeding the right breast and your right arm when breastfeeding the left breast. This position allows you to better guide your baby.

3-Soccer Ball Position:

You hold your baby under your armpit and stretch your baby's legs backwards. You can support your baby's head with your hand and guide it to your breast. This position can be comfortable for mothers who have had a caesarean section or mothers with large breasts.

4-Lying on your side:

Breastfeeding is done with the mother and baby lying side by side. The mother supports the baby with her lower arm and brings the baby's head closer to the nipple. This position is comfortable for night feedings.

Conclusion:

Breastfeeding contains antibodies that strengthen the baby's immune system and protect against diseases. The World Health Organization (WHO) recommends that babies are exclusively breastfed for the first six months. Breast milk contains all the necessary nutrients for the baby and is easy to digest.

It is important that the mother is relaxed and stress-free during breastfeeding. Stress can negatively affect milk production. Therefore, breastfeeding in a relaxed position and in a calm environment is beneficial for both mother and baby.

With the right techniques and positions, breastfeeding becomes a pleasant experience for both mother and baby. With this information, you can make your breastfeeding process more comfortable and efficient.

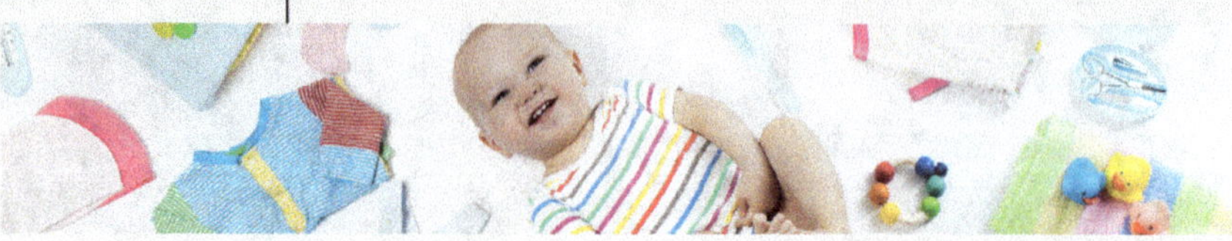

The care and sleep patterns of newborn babies is an important and demanding process for new parents. Proper care and sleep patterns play an important role in a baby's healthy development. Here are some scientific information and practical tips on this subject:

NEWBORN CARE
Newborn babies are delicate and vulnerable, so their care must be meticulous. Here are some basic care steps:

1-Nutrition:

-Breast Milk: Newborn babies usually need feeding every 2-3 hours. Breast milk is the ideal food because it strengthens the baby's immune system.

-Formula formula: If breast milk is not enough or breastfeeding is not possible, you can use formula. Choose the right formula for your baby in consultation with your doctor.

2-Hygiene:

-Bottom Changing: Change your baby's diaper often. Change the diaper every 2-3 hours or when it gets dirty.

-Navel Care: Keep this area clean and dry until the umbilical cord falls off. Wipe your baby clean with a sponge and leave the umbilical cord dry.

3-Clothing Selection:

-Cotton Clothes: Choose cotton clothes that do not irritate your baby's skin.

-Dressing according to the weather: Dress your baby according to the room temperature. Wear thin clothes in hot weather and layers in cold weather.

4-Touch and Attachment:

Skin-to-Skin Contact: Make frequent skin-to-skin contact with your baby. Hug, rock and soothe your baby. This reassures your baby and supports their emotional development.

-Eye Contact and Talking: Make eye contact with your baby and talk to him/her in a soft voice. This strengthens attachment.

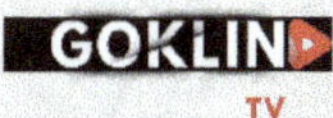

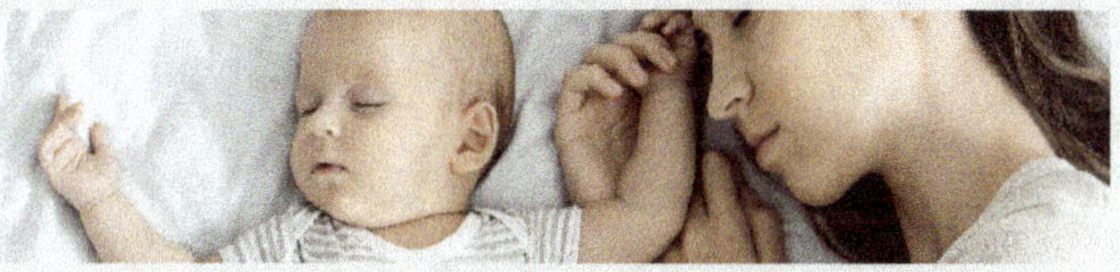

SLEEP PATTERN

Newborn babies can sleep 16-18 hours a day in the first few weeks, but sleep times can be short and irregular. You can follow these steps to establish a healthy sleep pattern:

1-Sleep Environment:

-Quiet and Dark Room: Make sure the room where your baby sleeps is quiet and dark. You can use a light night light.

-Crib Layout: Organize the crib with a firm mattress and tightly fitted sheets. Avoid soft pillows and toys.

2-Creating a Routine:

-Sleeping Routine: Establish a routine of going to sleep at the same time every night. For example, a warm bath, feeding and singing a lullaby. This routine signals to your baby that it is time to sleep.

-Separating Day and Night: Keep your baby bright and active during the day and feed and change at night in a quiet and dark environment. Thus, the baby learns the difference between day and night.

3-Sleeping on Your Own:

-Putting your baby to bed sleepy but awake: Put your baby in his/her crib when he/she is sleepy but still awake. This way he learns to fall asleep on his own.

-Night feedings: Keep night feeds as quiet and short as possible. This allows the baby to be fed without disturbing the sleep pattern.

4-Safety of the sleeping environment:

-Sleeping on your back: Always place your baby on his or her back. This is important to prevent sudden infant death syndrome (SIDS).

-Sleep Space Safety: The crib or cot should be safe and stable. Do not place pillows, stuffed toys or loose blankets in the baby's bed.

Meeting your baby's needs can sometimes be difficult, but be patient and adapt to their rhythm. Healthy care and a regular sleep routine are the cornerstones for your baby's physical and emotional development. Remember, every baby is different and will develop their own routine over time.

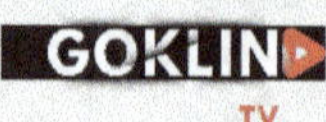

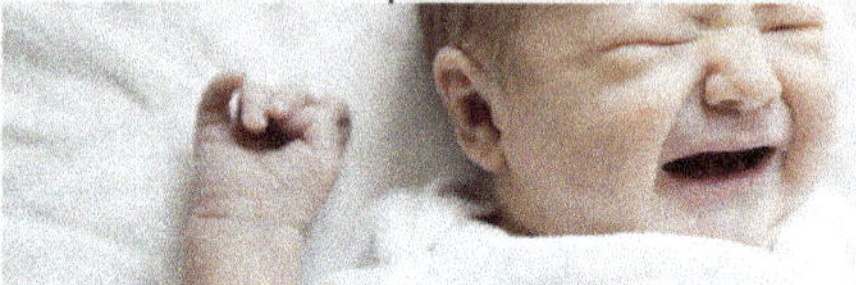

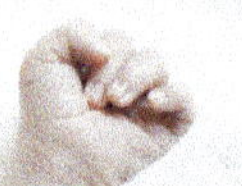

White noise is a type of continuous sound with a wide frequency spectrum. It is perceived by the human ear as a continuous "shhh" sound. Often, white noise machines or apps produce this sound and are used to help babies sleep.

BENEFİTS OF WHİTE NOİSE

1-Sleep Aid:

-Masking External Noise: White noise masks sudden and loud noises from the outside to help the baby fall asleep and prolong sleep. For example, traffic noise or other noises in the house.

-Mimics Womb Sounds: White noise is similar to the constant sounds a baby hears in the womb and can therefore be relaxing for the baby.

2-Relaxation and Calming:

-Reduces Stress and Anxiety: White noise can help babies relax and calm down. This can have a soothing effect, especially in colicky babies.

-Regular Sleep Habits: When used regularly, white noise can signal that it is time for a baby to go to sleep and can help establish sleep habits.

THE HARM OF WHİTE NOİSE

1-Risk of Addiction:

-Developing a habit: Your baby may get used to white noise and find it difficult to sleep without it. This can lead to your baby becoming addicted to white noise as they grow older.

2-Hearing Health:

-High Sound Levels: If a white noise machine or app is operated at high volume levels, it can damage a baby's hearing health. The American Academy of Pediatrics recommends that the sound level should not exceed 50 decibels.

-Prolonged Noise Exposure: Prolonged exposure to white noise can affect a baby's hearing and language development.

3-Safety Issues:

-Improper Use: White noise devices can create potential hazards when used incorrectly (for example, when placed too close to the baby or operated too loudly).

THİNGS TO CONSİDER WHEN USİNG WHİTE NOİSE

1-Volume Level: Keep the volume of the white noise device below 50 decibels. Place the device at least 2 meters away from your baby's crib.

2-Taking a Break: Instead of using the white noise device continuously, use it at regular intervals to prevent your baby from becoming addicted.

3-Monitoring Baby's Reactions: Monitor how your baby reacts to the white noise. If your baby does not relax or becomes uncomfortable with the white noise, stop using it.

Conclusion

White noise can be an effective tool to help newborn babies fall asleep and stay asleep. However, it is important to use it carefully and consciously. Controlling the volume, avoiding continuous use, and monitoring your baby's reactions can help you enjoy the benefits of white noise while avoiding the potential harms. Parents should discuss the use of white noise and other sleep management strategies with their doctor to determine the most appropriate approach.

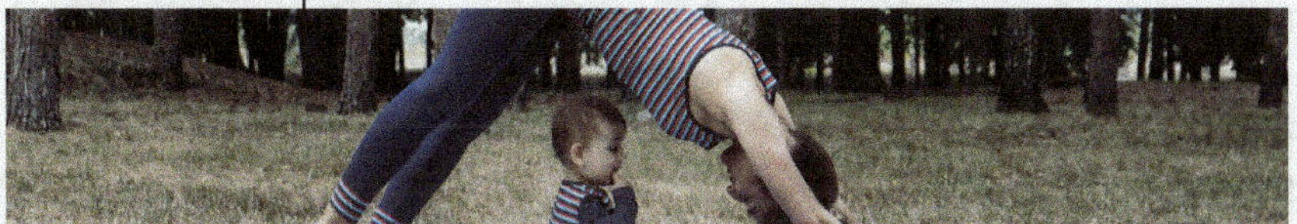

5-WHEN SHOULD POSTPARTUM EXERCİSES START?

Postnatal exercises are important to improve the mother's physical and mental health, increase energy levels and speed up the postpartum recovery process. However, the timing of when to start exercises depends on the mode of delivery, the mother's general health and the recovery process. Here's what you need to know about the process of starting postpartum exercises:

1. First week:
- After a normal vaginal delivery, light exercises can be started in the first week immediately after delivery. During this period, light activities such as walking and Kegel exercises to strengthen the pelvic floor muscles are recommended. These exercises promote healing by increasing blood circulation without overstraining the body.

2. First 6 Weeks:
- The first 6 weeks after birth is a time when the body should focus on the natural healing process. This process is especially important for mothers who gave birth by caesarean section. Intense exercise should be avoided during the first 6 weeks. Light walks, slow-paced yoga and gentle stretching can be done.

3. After the 6th Week:
- More intense exercises can be started 6 weeks after birth with the approval of the doctor. During this period, activities such as light abdominal exercises, swimming, low-impact aerobic exercises and yoga can be done to strengthen the abdominal muscles. However, the intensity of the exercises should be increased gradually and the body should rest.

4. Listen to Body Signals:
- It is important to listen to your body's signals when starting exercises. If you feel excessive fatigue, pain or discomfort, you should reduce or stop the exercises. In addition, breastfeeding mothers should drink plenty of water after exercise and ensure adequate nutritional intake.

5. Kegel Exercises:
- Kegel exercises help strengthen the pelvic floor muscles after childbirth. These exercises can help prevent postpartum problems such as urinary incontinence and pelvic organ prolapse. Doing Kegel exercises several times a day is an important step in the postpartum period.

Sample Exercise Plan:
- **First Week:** Light walks and Kegel exercises for 10-15 minutes a day.
- **First 6 Weeks:** 20-30 minute walks a day, light yoga and stretching.
- **After Week 6:** Low-impact aerobic exercises, abdominal exercises and swimming 3-4 times a week.

Conclusion:
When to start postpartum exercises depends on the mother's recovery and the doctor's recommendations. Mothers who have had a normal delivery can usually start light exercise from the first week, while mothers who have had a caesarean section may take a little longer. During the first 6 weeks, it is important to do light activities and allow the body to heal. After 6 weeks, more intense exercises can be started with the doctor's approval. Listening to your body and gradually increasing exercises will help you have a healthy postpartum period.

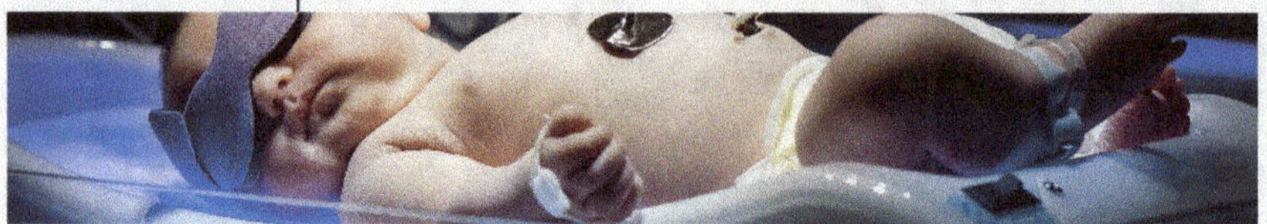

Neonatal jaundice is a common condition in babies in the first weeks after birth. Jaundice is characterized by the baby's skin and whites of the eyes turning yellow. This is caused by high levels of a substance called bilirubin in the blood. Here are the causes of jaundice in newborn babies:

1. What is bilirubin?
- Bilirubin is a substance formed as a result of the breakdown of red blood cells. It is normally processed by the liver and excreted from the body. However, because the liver of newborn babies is not yet fully mature, it cannot process bilirubin fast enough, causing its level in the blood to rise.

2. Types of Neonatal Jaundice:
- **Physiologic Jaundice:** It is the most common type and usually starts on the second or third day of life. It occurs because the baby's liver cannot process bilirubin fast enough. It usually does not require treatment and resolves spontaneously within a few weeks.

- **Breast Milk Jaundice:** It can be seen in babies who are breastfed. Some substances in breast milk can slow down the processing of bilirubin by the liver. It is usually harmless and continued breastfeeding is recommended.

- **Pathologic Jaundice:** This is more serious and can be caused by various health problems. It can be caused by blood group incompatibility, infections or congenital liver diseases. It requires rapid medical intervention.

3. Symptoms of jaundice:
- Yellowing of the skin and whites of the eyes is the most obvious symptom. The baby may also show signs of weakness, difficulty sucking and restlessness. If the jaundice spreads to the baby's abdomen and legs, this may be a sign of a more serious problem.

4. Treatment of jaundice:
- **Phototherapy:** This is known as light therapy. The baby is held under a special light, which helps the body to process bilirubin more easily.

- **Breast milk and nutrition:** Frequent breastfeeding can help remove bilirubin from the body. If the baby is not getting enough nutrition, it can be supplemented with formula.

- **Blood Changes:** With very high bilirubin levels, a blood transfusion may be necessary. This is reserved for rare and serious cases.

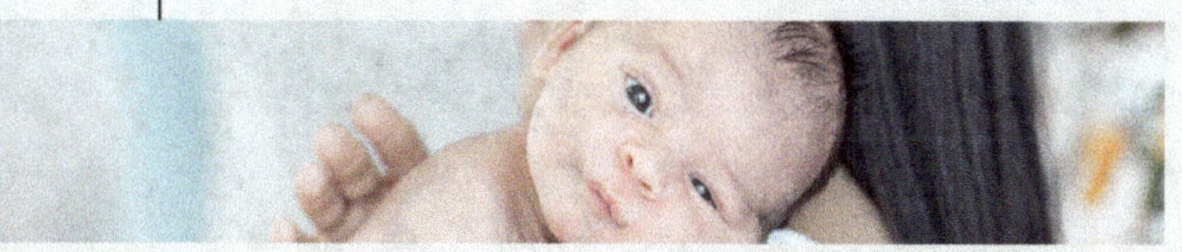

Gas pains in babies are a common occurrence for new parents and a common cause of baby restlessness. Gas pains are caused by the immaturity of a baby's digestive system and usually occur in the first few months of life. Here are some methods that can be used to relieve gas pains in babies:

1. Correct Breastfeeding and Feeding Technique:

- It is important to feed in the correct position to prevent the baby from swallowing too much air during breastfeeding or bottle feeding. The baby's head and torso should be aligned and the baby should be able to fully grasp the breast or bottle tip. When bottle feeding, it should be preferred that the bottle has an airtight design.

2. Frequent Burping:

- The baby should burp frequently during or after feeding. This helps expel air bubbles in the stomach. Gently patting the baby on the back by leaning the baby on your shoulder or lying face down on your lap can help the baby burp.

3. Abdominal massage:

- Gently massaging the baby's tummy can relieve gas pains. While the baby is lying on his/her back, massaging the abdomen with clockwise circular movements can facilitate the passage of gas through the intestines.

4. Warm Applications:

- Putting a warm diaper on the baby's tummy can relieve gas pains. Warming the baby's tummy with a warm washcloth or a hot water bottle can relax the muscles and facilitate the expulsion of gas.

*****NOTE: Avoid putting a hot water bottle or diaper directly on the baby's skin. Wrap the diaper or bag in a washcloth or towel before putting it on the baby's skin. This prevents direct heat contact and reduces the risk of burns.

5. Movement and Position Changes:

- Moving babies and changing their position can encourage gas to move through the intestines. Gently rocking the baby on your lap or doing bicycle movements (moving the baby's legs as if pedaling gently) can relieve gas pains.

6. Probiotics:

- Some research shows that probiotic supplements can reduce gas pains in babies. However, a doctor should be consulted about the use of probiotics.

Conclusion:

Gas pains in babies are usually caused by the immaturity of their digestive system and can be alleviated with a few simple methods. Proper breastfeeding and feeding techniques, frequent burping, abdominal massage, warm applications and movement can be effective in reducing gas pains. Probiotic supplements can also help, but a doctor should be consulted. These methods help the baby to relax and the parents to get through this process more easily.

8-WHAT CAN BE DONE TO İNCREASE BREAST MİLK?

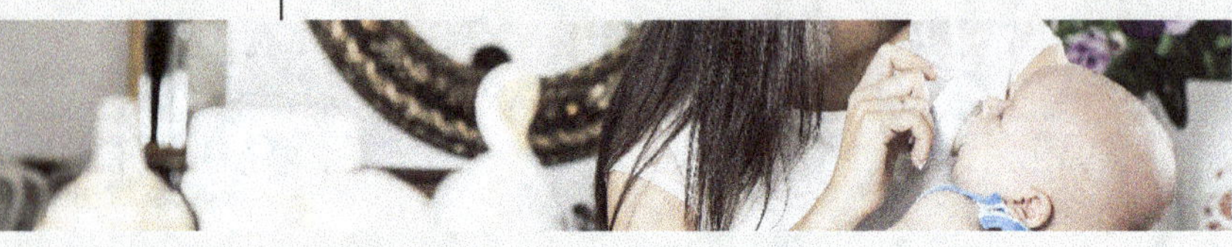

Breast milk is the most valuable source of nutrition for newborn babies and plays a critical role in their healthy growth and development. However, some mothers may worry about not producing enough milk. There are some scientifically supported methods to increase breast milk. Here's what can be done to increase breast milk and why:

1. Breastfeeding Frequently:
- Frequent breastfeeding provides continuous stimulation of the mammary glands. The hormones prolactin and oxytocin are secreted during breastfeeding. Prolactin stimulates milk production, while oxytocin causes the milk ducts to contract and milk is released.

2. Correct Breastfeeding Technique:
- When the baby latches on to the breast correctly and sucks effectively, milk production increases. Incorrect breastfeeding techniques can cause sores on the nipples and reduced milk production. Correct breastfeeding positions and techniques ensure that the baby gets enough milk and help the mammary glands to empty effectively.

3. Drink plenty of fluids:
- Breast milk is largely made up of water. Adequate fluid intake is essential for the body to maintain milk production. Drinking enough water maintains the body's hydration level and supports milk production.

4. Balanced and Nutritious Diet:
- It is important for nursing mothers to consume foods rich in protein, vitamins and minerals. Especially foods containing omega-3 fatty acids and iron support milk production. Adequate nutrient intake provides the body with the energy needed for milk production.

5. Reducing Stress:
- Stress can negatively affect milk production. High levels of the stress hormone cortisol suppress milk production. Stress management techniques such as relaxing activities, meditation and yoga can increase milk production.

6. Breastfeeding Support and Pumping:
- Using a milk pump between feedings can increase milk production. Pumping provides continuous stimulation of the mammary glands and encourages milk production. In addition, receiving breastfeeding counseling ensures the correct application of techniques and positively affects milk production.

9-WHAT ARE POSTPARTUM WEİGHT LOSS METHODS?

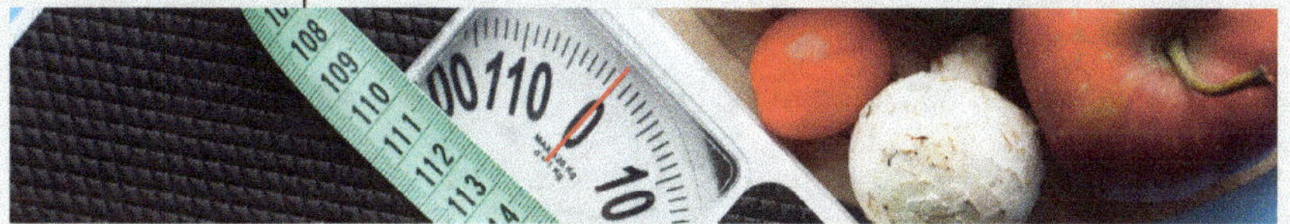

Losing weight after childbirth is one of the most common issues that new mothers face. Losing the weight gained during pregnancy in a healthy way is important for both the physical and psychological well-being of the mother. Here are some effective methods that can help with postpartum weight loss:

Balanced and Nutritious Diet: A balanced diet is the cornerstone of weight loss. Consuming foods rich in protein, fiber, vitamins and minerals not only improves breast milk quality but also helps with weight loss. For example, eating eggs for breakfast meets your protein needs and helps you stay full for a long time. For lunch and dinner, you can choose salads with lots of vegetables and grilled chicken or fish. It is important to avoid processed foods, sugary drinks and high-calorie snacks.

Regular Exercise: Physical activity is an effective way to burn calories and boost metabolism. Light walks, yoga, pilates and postnatal exercise programs can help mothers get in shape safely. Brisk walks of 30 minutes a day increase your body's energy expenditure and facilitate weight loss.

Adequate Sleep: Inadequate sleep can contribute to weight gain and make it harder to lose weight. It can be difficult for new moms to establish a sleeping pattern, but it is important to try to get as much rest as possible. Getting enough sleep balances your metabolism and makes it easier to control weight.

Drink plenty of water: Water is essential for the proper functioning of the metabolism and increases the feeling of fullness, reducing the desire to overeat. You can drink a glass of water before each meal to increase your daily water consumption. Also, adequate hydration during breastfeeding supports milk production and makes it easier for you to lose weight.

Breastfeeding: Breastfeeding helps the mother's body burn calories and makes the uterus shrink faster. Breastfeeding mothers can burn up to 500 extra calories per day. Therefore, breastfeeding offers many benefits not only for the baby but also for the mother.

Sample Diet Plan
- **Morning Breakfast:** 2 boiled eggs, whole wheat bread, tomato, cucumber
- **Snack:** Handful of walnuts or almonds
- **Lunch:** Grilled chicken, salad with lots of greens
- **Snack:** Yogurt and one fruit
- **Dinner:** Grilled fish, steamed vegetables
- **Night Snack:** Herbal tea and a slice of cheese

By following these methods, you can lose weight in a healthy way after giving birth and maintain your overall health. Remember, losing weight can take time and it is important to be patient.

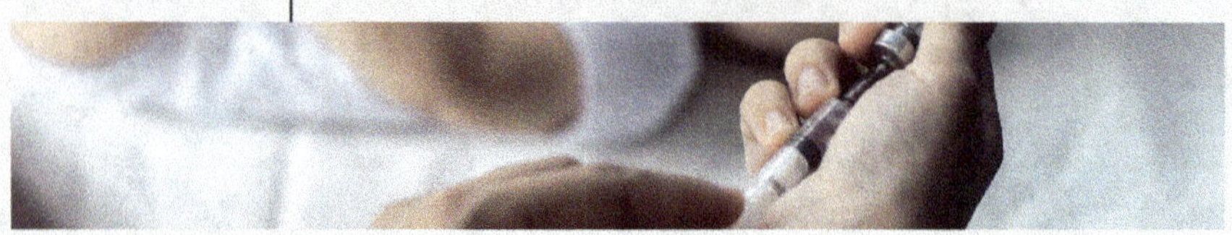

It is very important that babies are vaccinated regularly so that they grow up healthy. Vaccinations protect babies from many serious diseases and strengthen their immune systems. Following the vaccination schedule correctly is an important issue that parents should pay attention to. Here is a guide on how to keep track of your baby's vaccination schedule and a sample schedule:

1. Importance of the Immunization Schedule: Vaccines protect babies from diphtheria, tetanus, whooping cough, measles, mumps, rubella, hepatitis B, polio, tuberculosis and many other diseases. The World Health Organization (WHO) and the Ministry of Health determine the recommended vaccination schedule for babies. This calendar shows which vaccines babies should receive at which ages and is updated regularly by health professionals.

2. Keeping track of the vaccination schedule: To keep track of the vaccination schedule, it is useful to keep a vaccination card or notebook from the moment your baby is born. You can get information about the vaccination schedule from health centers, hospitals or family doctors and update this card each time you receive a vaccine.

Things to Consider When Keeping Track of Vaccinations:
- **Don't Miss Appointments:** Vaccinations should be given at certain times. Take care not to miss your appointments and, if necessary, contact your healthcare provider to get reminders.
- **Be Aware of Side Effects:** Vaccines can often have mild side effects. Ask health professionals about these side effects and be prepared for possible situations.
- **Communicate with the Doctor:** Consult your doctor if you have any questions or concerns.

Possible Side Effects of Vaccines
Vaccines are generally safe and serious side effects are rare. However, some babies may experience mild side effects.

- **Redness or swelling at the vaccination site:** There may be mild redness or swelling at the vaccination site. This usually goes away within a few days.
- **Mild Fever:** Babies may have a mild fever after vaccination. This is a sign that the immune system is responding and is usually short-lived.
- **Restlessness and crankiness:** Babies may become restless and cranky after vaccination. This is usually short-lived.
- **Loss of appetite:** Some babies may experience loss of appetite after vaccination.
- **Changes in Sleep Patterns:** Babies may have temporary changes in their sleep patterns after vaccination.

10-HOW TO FOLLOW THE INFANT VACCİNATİON SCHEDULE?

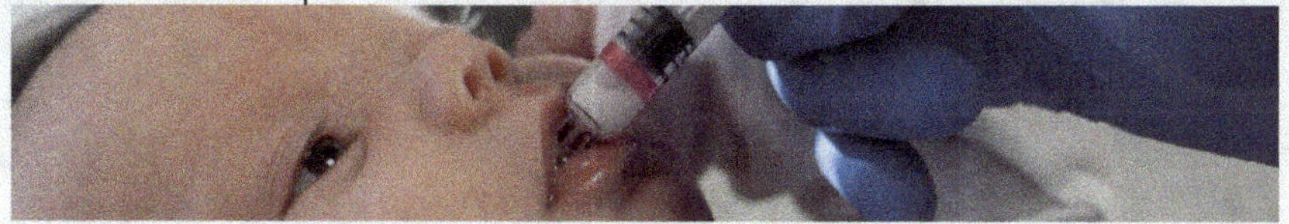

SAMPLE INFANT IMMUNİZATİON SCHEDULE TRACKİNG PLAN

At birth
- **Hepatitis B vaccine (1st dose)**

1st month:
Hepatitis B vaccine (2nd dose)

2nd month:
- **Diphtheria, Tetanus, Pertussis (DaBT-IPA-Hib) vaccine (1st dose)**
- **Polio (polio) vaccine (1st dose)**
- **Pneumococcal (pneumonia) vaccine (1st dose)**
- **Rotavirus vaccine (1st dose)**

4th month:
- **Diphtheria, Tetanus, Pertussis (DaBT-IPA-Hib) vaccine (2nd dose)**
- **Polio (polio) vaccine (2nd dose)**
- **Pneumococcal (pneumonia) vaccine (2nd dose)**
- **Rotavirus vaccine (2nd dose)**

6th month:
- **Diphtheria, Tetanus, Pertussis (DaBT-IPA-Hib) vaccine (3rd dose)**
- **Polio (polio) vaccine (3rd dose)**
- **Hepatitis B vaccine (3rd dose)**

12th month:
- **Measles, Mumps, Rubella (MMR) vaccine (1st dose)**
- **Pneumococcal (pneumonia) vaccine (booster dose)**
- **Hepatitis A vaccine (1st dose)**

18th month:
- **Diphtheria, Tetanus, Pertussis (DaBT-IPA-Hib) vaccine (booster dose)**
- **Hepatitis A vaccine (2nd dose)**

24th month and later:
- **Measles, Mumps, Rubella (MMR) vaccine (2nd dose)**
- **Meningitis vaccine**

This sample plan will help you understand how to follow the immunization schedule so that babies grow up healthy. Be sure to get detailed and up-to-date information from your health care provider or doctor.

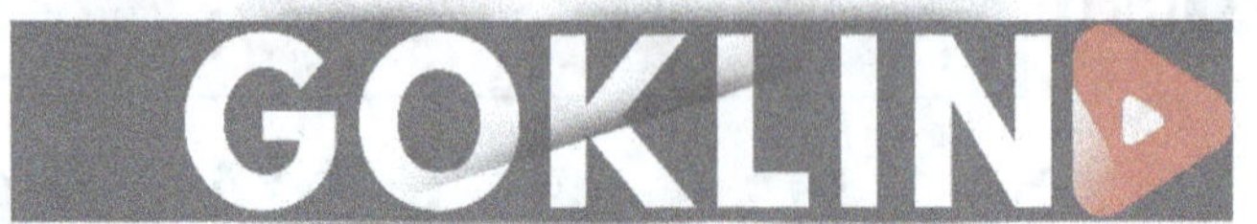

PREGNANCY CALENDAR AND CHECKLIST

1ST TRİMESTER (WEEKS 1-13)

Week	Fetal Development	Health Check-ups	Notes and Tips	Completed (✓)
1	Fertilization and implantation occur		Adopt a healthy lifestyle	
2	Fertilized egg implants in the uterus			
3	Embryo development begins			
4	Hormone levels rise, pregnancy symptoms may appear	Plan first doctor's appointment	Adopt a healthy diet and lifestyle	
5	Heartbeat can be heard			
6	Brain and spinal cord begin to develop			
7	Eyes and nose start to form			
8	Fingers and fingertips become more defined	First ultrasound		
9	Organs start to develop			
10	Kidneys, liver, and brain development accelerates			
11	Gender starts to become distinguishable		First trimester screening and blood tests	
12	Nails and hair start to develop			
13	Rapid fetal growth, facial features become clearer		Start wearing comfortable clothes	

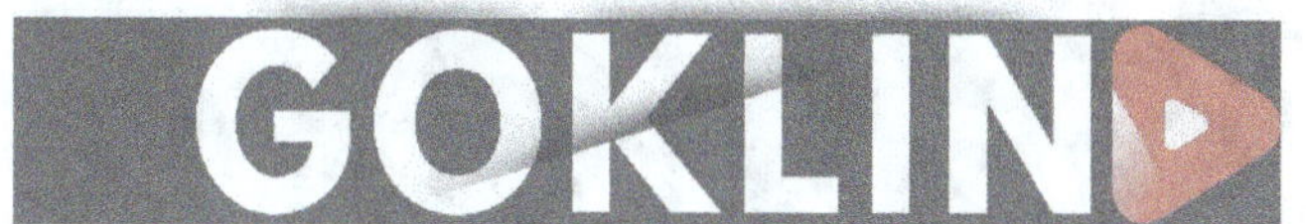

TV

PREGNANCY CALENDAR AND CHECKLIST

2ND TRİMESTER (WEEKS 14-26)

Week	Fetal Development	Health Check-ups	Notes and Tips	Completed (✓)
14	Baby's movements may be felt		Continue a balanced diet	
15	Bones start to harden			
16	Baby can hear sounds			
17	Fat tissue develops			
18	Ears fully develop	Detailed ultrasound, anomaly screening	Review birth plan	
19	Nervous system develops			
20	Baby establishes sleep patterns			
21	Baby's movements become more pronounced			
22	Taste buds develop			
23	Lungs begin to develop			
24	Baby starts to gain weight	Gestational diabetes test		
25	Spine development continues			
26	Lungs continue to mature		Choose comfortable clothing	

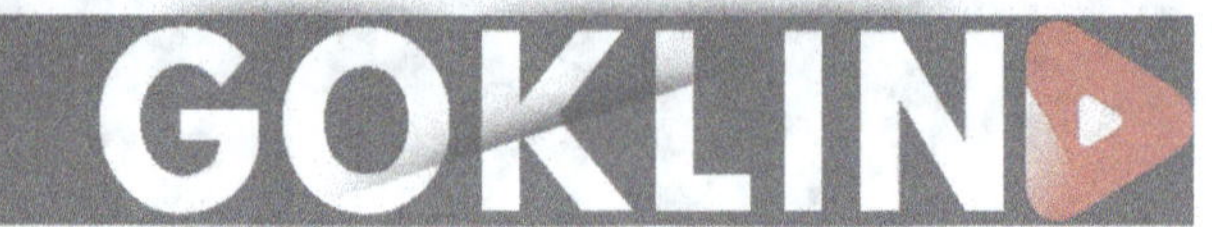

PREGNANCY CALENDAR AND CHECKLIST
3RD TRİMESTER (WEEKS 27-40)

Week	Fetal Development	Health Check-ups	Notes and Tips	Completed (✓)
27	Baby grows rapidly	Regular doctor visits, blood pressure, and urine tests	Attend childbirth classes	
28	Brain development speeds up	Rh immunoglobulin (for Rh-negative mothers)		
29	Baby can open and close eyes			
30	Bones are fully developed			
31	Baby experiences sleep and wake cycles		Prepare hospital bag	
32	Skin becomes pink and smooth			
33	Lungs are fully developed			
34	Baby continues to gain weight			
35	Baby's position is checked, NST test may be performed	Group B strep test	Watch for labor signs	
36	Baby may be in a head-down position			
37	Baby prepares for birth			
38	Baby is ready for birth, continues to gain weight			
39	Monitor baby's movements		Stay in touch with the hospital	
40	Labor begins			

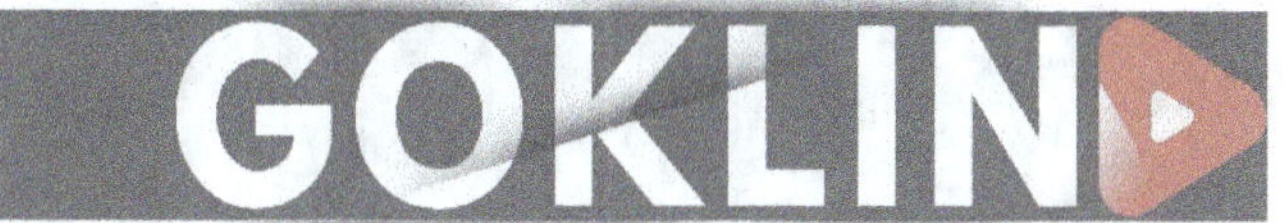

SPECİAL NOTES:

- **Weeks 4-12: First Trimester Tests:** During the first trimester, you will undergo several initial tests including blood tests and ultrasounds to confirm the pregnancy and assess the initial development of the fetus. These tests help in detecting any early potential complications and ensuring the pregnancy is progressing normally.

- **Weeks 16-18: Quadruple Test:** The quadruple test, or quad screen, is a blood test that measures four specific substances in the mother's blood. It helps to assess the risk of the baby having certain genetic conditions such as Down syndrome, trisomy 18, and neural tube defects.

- **Week 20: Detailed Ultrasound:** Also known as the anatomy scan, this ultrasound provides a detailed view of the baby's organs and structures. It helps to ensure that the baby is developing properly and can identify any physical abnormalities.

- **Weeks 24-28: Gestational Diabetes Screening:** This test checks for gestational diabetes, a type of diabetes that develops during pregnancy. It involves drinking a glucose solution and having your blood sugar levels tested an hour later. If the results are high, further testing may be needed.

- **Week 28: Rh Immunoglobulin:** If you have Rh-negative blood, you will receive an Rh immunoglobulin injection to prevent your immune system from attacking the baby's Rh-positive blood cells, which can lead to complications.

- **Weeks 35-37: Group B Strep Test:** This test checks for Group B Streptococcus (GBS) bacteria in the vagina and rectum. If GBS is present, antibiotics will be given during labor to prevent the baby from getting infected during delivery.

These detailed special notes provide crucial information on what to expect and the significance of each test and check-up throughout the pregnancy.

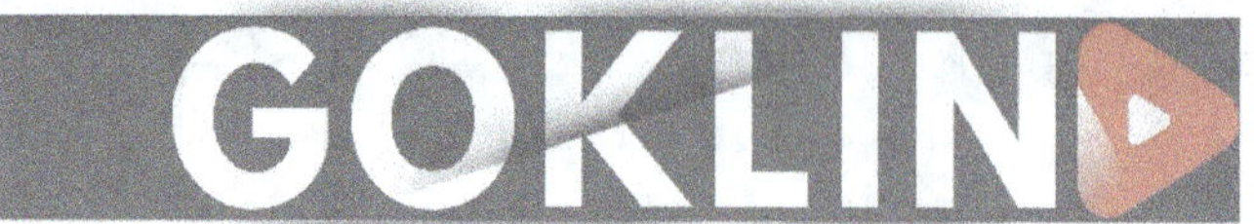

BETA HCG AND WHEN YOUR BODY STARTS PRODUCING HCG

What is Beta hCG?

Beta hCG (human chorionic gonadotropin) is a hormone produced by the placenta during the early stages of pregnancy. Pregnancy tests detect the presence of this hormone. Beta hCG is produced after the embryo implants in the uterus and its levels continue to rise throughout pregnancy.

When Does Your Body Start Producing hCG?

Your body starts producing hCG approximately 6-12 days after fertilization. During this period, the fertilized egg implants in the uterus and the placenta begins to develop. hCG levels rise rapidly during the first weeks of pregnancy and reach their peak around the 10th week. Thereafter, they stabilize during the second trimester and continue at this level until birth.

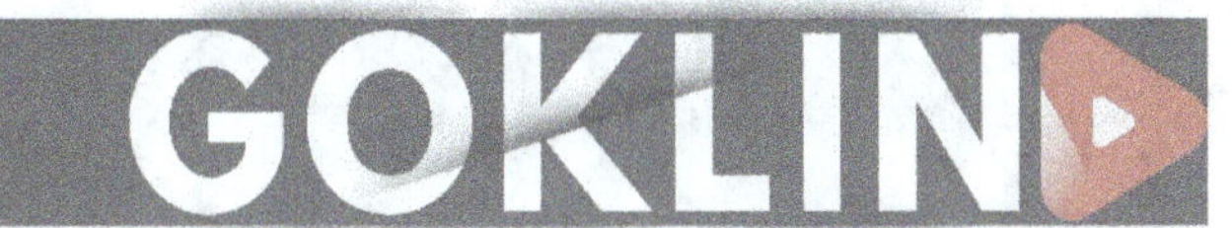

TV

HCG LEVELS AND TİMELİNE

Gestational Week	hCG Levels (mIU/mL)
3	5 - 50
4	5 - 426
5	18 - 7,340
6	1,080 - 56,500
7-8	7,650 - 229,000
9-12	25,700 - 288,000
13-16	13,300 - 254,000
17-24	4,060 - 165,400
25-40	3,640 - 117,000

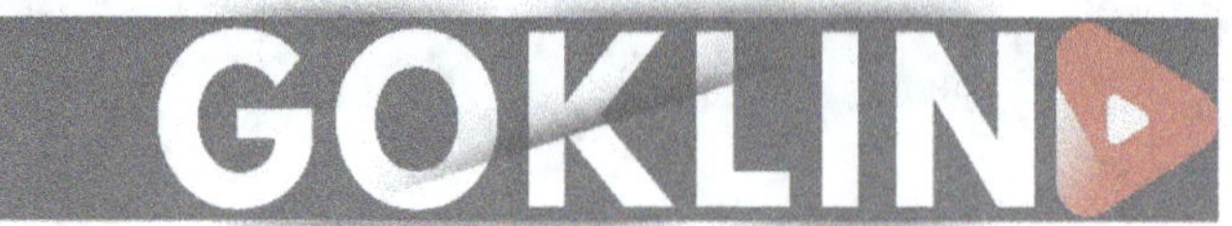

HCG LEVELS AND TİMELİNE

0-2 Weeks: Ovulation and fertilization.

2-4 Weeks: The fertilized egg implants in the uterus and the placenta begins to develop. hCG production starts.

4-10 Weeks: hCG levels rise rapidly.

10-12 Weeks: hCG levels reach their peak.

12-24 Weeks: hCG levels stabilize.

24-40 Weeks: hCG levels remain constant and continue until birth.

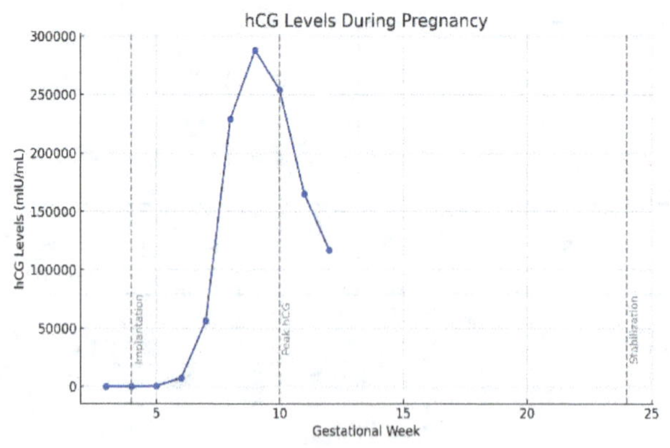

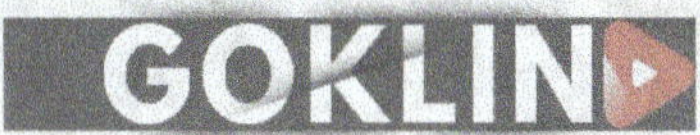

TV

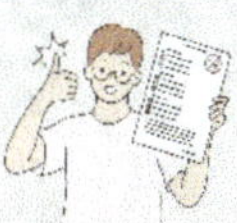
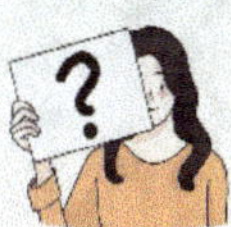

DAD-TO-BE READİNESS QUİZ: 'AM I READY FOR FATHERHOOD?'

Becoming a father is a huge responsibility and one of life's most exciting adventures. But how ready are you for this journey? To ensure you can support your partner during pregnancy and beyond, why not take this fun 15-question quiz? Each 'Yes' answer indicates you're one step closer to being ready for fatherhood, while each 'No' answer highlights an area that might need a bit more consideration. Let's see, dads-to-be, how ready are you for this fatherhood adventure?

1-Are you and your partner on the same page about having children?
Yes / No

2-Are you prepared to share baby care and household chores?
Yes / No

3-Do you think you can handle stressful and sleepless nights?
Yes / No

4-Have you adjusted your financial situation to accommodate having a baby?
Yes / No

5-Have you done any education or research on parenting?
Yes / No

6-Do you know how to support your partner during pregnancy and childbirth?
Yes / No

7-Are you ready for the lifestyle changes that come with having a baby?
Yes / No

8-Are you satisfied with your own fatherhood role model?
Yes / No

9-Do you have basic principles for child-rearing, and do you share them with your partner?
Yes / No

10-Have you considered taking leave from work or adjusting your work schedule to spend time with the baby?
Yes / No

11-Have you thought about how having a child will affect your social life?
Yes / No

12-Have you made necessary financial arrangements for health insurance and baby care?
Yes / No

13-Have you thought about how having a baby will impact your relationship with your partner?
Yes / No

14-Are you ready to put off personal goals and hobbies to fulfill parenting responsibilities?
Yes / No

15-Do you have a support network of family or friends to help with parenting?
Yes / No

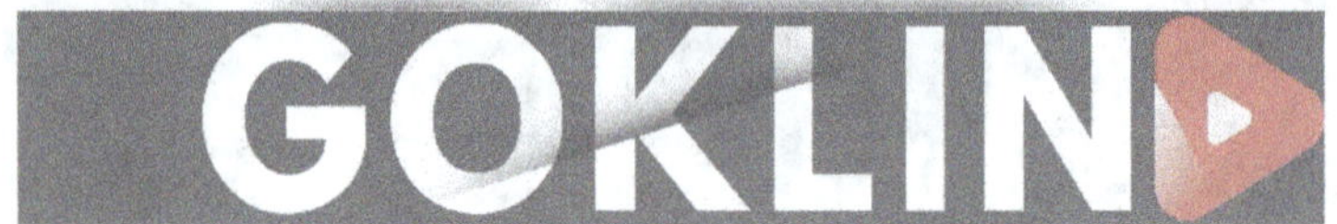

Dear Readers

"Pregnancy Secrets: 50 Striking Questions and Answers for Every Stage" has come to an end. I hope this book has shed light on every stage you have experienced or will experience before, during and after pregnancy. We are happy if you have found answers to the questions that have been on your mind throughout your journey!

Our aim in writing this book was to make every step of the pregnancy process more understandable and easier for you. Sometimes the answer to one question can be enough to clear the confusion in our minds. In choosing these 50 questions for you, we have taken care to cover the most curious and critical topics.

Remember, every pregnancy and birth process is unique. Your own body and your doctor will be your greatest guides during this process. We wish you a healthy, peaceful and happy pregnancy.

Finally, don't forget to visit our GöklinTV social media page for more information and up-to-date content. We are waiting for you there too!

Stay with love and health,
GöklinTV

www.ingramcontent.com/pod-product-compliance
Lightning Source LLC
Chambersburg PA
CBHW070801250726
48662CB00004B/1921